Scribe Publications
HEADACHE

Dr Carole Hungerford became a general practitioner in 1975. After working for five years in London, she has for the last 20 years shared her time between her rural practice in Bathurst, New South Wales, and her practice in eastern Sydney. She has helped educate young graduates for the Royal Australian College of General Practitioners, and she is also a fellow of the Australasian College of Nutritional and Environmental Medicine. Her previous book is *Good Health in the 21st Century*, which won the Science Writing Award in the 2006 Queensland Premier's Literary Awards. Carole's website is www.carolehungerford.com.

HEADACHE

A family doctor's guide
to treating a common ailment

Dr CAROLE HUNGERFORD

SCRIBE
Melbourne · London

Scribe Publications Pty Ltd
18–20 Edward St, Brunswick, Victoria 3056, Australia
50A Kingsway Place, Sans Walk, London, EC1R 0LU, United Kingdom

First published by Scribe 2014

Typeset in 11.5/16 pt Goudy Old Style by the publishers
Printed and bound in Australia by Griffin Press

The paper this book is printed on is certified against the Forest
Stewardship Council® Standards. Griffin Press holds FSC chain
of custody certification SGS-COC-005088. FSC promotes
environmentally responsible, socially beneficial and economically
viable management of the world's forests.

National Library of Australia
Cataloguing-in-Publication data

Hungerford, Carole, author.

Headache / by Carole Hungerford.

9781922070470 (Australian edition)
9781922247759 (UK edition)
9781925113006 (e-book)

1. Headache. 2. Migraine.

616.8491

scribepublications.com.au
scribepublications.co.uk

Contents

Introduction

'At one time, people thought that migraine was a disorder all its own and that tension-type headache was totally separate. Now we know that headaches are not all that clear cut.'
DOCTOR NINAN MATHEW

This book is all about headache. It is not about the medical emergencies, often referred to as 'secondary' headaches, that present in the emergency department. It is about the headaches that the family doctor sees every day. It is about the headaches that rob individuals of quality of life, and the nation of time lost from work. We regard such headaches as 'primary' headaches.

The spectrum of people who get headaches is wide; it is not easy to predict who will suffer from them. At one extreme are the hardy souls — by no means few in number — who can barely remember ever having had a headache. The US National Institute of Neurological Disorders and Stroke have evidence that 10 per cent of men and 5 per cent of women don't have a single headache during their entire lives.[1] At the other extreme are those whose lives are dominated by headache. And in between there is a lot of variation concerning who gets headaches and how often they get them.

Clearly headache is more than one illness, and it afflicts more than one personality type.

What we do know is that the size of the problem is growing. In this, the second decade of the millennium, it is estimated that approximately 45 million Americans get chronic headache. That's about one in six people. Of these headaches, 28 million are classified as 'migraine'. The rest are due to the other causes.[2] In the United Kingdom, about 6 million adults suffer from migraine. On any one day, 200,000 people will experience a migraine. Half of them will miss school or work. The cost to the National Health Service for medications and visits to the doctor is estimated at £150 million a year. In terms of time lost from work, the estimate of cost to the UK economy is £2.25 billion, with 5 million working weeks lost each year. Added to this, of course, are the days lost to work as the result of headaches not classified as 'migraine'.[3] In Australia, while no major studies have been undertaken, it is estimated that there are more than 3 million migraine sufferers and more than 7 million sufferers of tension headaches. Twenty-three per cent of households contain at least one migraine sufferer, and the direct and indirect costs of migraine are estimated to be around $1 billion annually.[4]

The World Health Organization has placed migraine among the world's 20 leading causes of disability.[5] Chronic headaches from other causes simply add to this.

Why are headaches growing in number? Is it that we are exposed to more chemicals than in the past, or that we are eating more processed foods, or that we are working longer hours — or a combination of all of these things? We do not yet know the answer, but we do know that it will continue to cost individuals, doctors, and even nations both time and money as people continue to suffer.

This book is not about me, but it would be disingenuous not to tell the story that I know best of all. This book discusses other case histories, using pseudonyms and changing some biographical details to preserve anonymity. I have no such restrictions on my own story.

I am a sufferer of migraine, although it took me many years to realise the full implications of this, and to see the pattern to my headaches.

As a child, I suffered from car sickness, often when my grandmother was in the car. She would sit in the back between my brother and me, and slip us chocolate when our mother was not looking. (There were rules about sweets, which Nanna treated with grandmotherly disdain.) Nanna also wore perfume, with which I had a love–hate relationship. On the one hand, it smelled exotic and pretty; on the other, it gave me a sick feeling, which I would now identify as a migraine aura.

At the age of nine, I had my first experience of migraine. I felt a pain around my face so distinct that you could draw a line around it. I had a dull headache on top of my head, and mild nausea. Once again, poor Nanna was unwittingly the cause. She had given me my first mango. The smell and flavour was sickly sweet and yet enticing, both at the same time. (I probably got some chocolate also.) I ate the fruit, but asked if the mangoes could be kept in another room because I found their smell unpleasant.

A few years later, when I was in high school and just entering puberty, I woke one night and was unable to get back to sleep. My father, who was still up, offered me some rum and milk, his own cure for insomnia (and just about everything else). I went back to sleep quite quickly, but at school the following day. I remember telling my teacher about the peculiar headache I was experiencing. It was all over one side of my head, and again I noticed that the edge of it was sharply defined, as if I could trace a line along the border.

After that, I had a few more migrainous events — headaches with features such as visual disturbance, but that stopped short of anything that would be classified as a full-blown migraine. Several times they occurred after eating cashew nuts. I was a serious competitive swimmer, and I began to notice another interesting symptom. As the swimming season wore on and the water got colder, I was developing Raynaud's phenomenon. When I was cold, the tips of all of my fingers would become white and bloodless, and eventually this would extend to the entire length of the outer two fingers. I also developed painful chilblains in my toes. Sensitivity to cold, leading to spasm in the tiny blood vessels of the fingers and toes, has a recognised connection to some forms of headache, but of course I did not know that then.

Once I entered medical school, the headaches became more frequent, although they were still reasonably rare. Various things would set them off. Sitting under a flickering fluorescent light in the library was intolerable. Eating dark chocolate or oranges, or drinking red wine, was a disaster.

Eating peanuts and cashew nuts was almost as bad. Then, one day, on my way to an exam, I splashed perfume all over myself to put me in a positive mood for the exam. The result was nearly catastrophic. I fought nausea, and had trouble making sense of words in the questions, which ran into one another. I fear that many of my answers must have looked like babble to the examiners. I did get through the exam, but I will never know how.

So over time and through experience I learned what to avoid, what triggered a headache. And yet I was often still caught out. Some of the occurrences were 'Friday-night headaches', where the adrenalin rush of the week somehow kept the headache at bay, only for it to declare itself when the pressure came off. But what about the rest of the time?

Then came my first pregnancy, and with it 'morning sickness' that lasted all day. My enlightened profession, dizzy with psychoanalytic enthusiasm, was in the habit of describing this as an 'unconscious rejection of the baby'. By the second and third pregnancies, doctors knew more, and it was diagnosed as *hyperemesis gravidarum*, or excessive vomiting during pregnancy. (Charlotte Brontë's death is believed to have been caused by *hyperemesis gravidarum*, and it is sad to note that Brontë's friend, Mrs Gaskell, wrote of her that even before the pregnancy, 'indigestion, nausea, headache, sleeplessness ... all combined to produce miserable depression of spirits'.)

I did not make a link then between my headaches and pregnancy sickness. It was a couple of decades after my pregnancies, and about a century too late for Brontë, before migraine was seriously listed as a risk for *hyperemesis*. From where I stand now, this was one of the many pieces that have come together in the puzzle of headaches.

Some time after the birth of my children, and long before the advent of the genetic information we will be discussing shortly, a chance encounter with a cousin, a fellow migraineur, led me to consult Robert Buist, PhD. Steeped in an understanding of immunology and biochemistry, he set me on a dietary path that resolved my headaches and transformed the way I practised medicine. He was the first clinician that I had met who made any scientific link between diet and health symptoms. He basically put the solution into my hands.

Robert Buist's books appear in the further reading section, and this book is dedicated to him in gratitude.

In the past, there was a social stigma attached to someone who always seemed to be suffering from a headache. And if I am to be very honest, this is still often the case. It would seem that someone who is getting more than an 'average' number of headaches is viewed with suspicion.

Why is this? Is it because symptoms are not visible, often even to the professional eye? Or is it that we measure other people's health against our own? If *we* can work long hours, stare at a computer screen all day, skip lunch, and still not develop a headache, why can't others?

Fortunately, this is changing as we gather more information about headaches. For one, we can now use brain imaging with MRI during, for example, a migraine, and get a picture of what is going on inside the head. Genetic studies are throwing up all sorts of clues as to who gets headaches and why. Chemical sensitivity is often linked to headache, and we now know a lot more about the genetic link to this as well. With this knowledge comes the possibility of answers.

In this book I identify some of the events or actions that can set us, unknowingly, on the path to the headaches that dominate lives. And I present some ideas I have gathered, both from the science and from the patients I have seen along the way.

But this is not a neurology textbook. It is aimed at readers afflicted by headaches, who want options to deal with them. I will look at some of the basic science of headaches, and discuss ways of getting relief beyond, but not necessarily excluding, prescription medicines. Medication has its part to play, but I think it is a mistake to see it as our only weapon. I am writing for those people who feel that *something* might be contributing to their headaches, but they just can't nail what. Some of the simple things I will explore are practices an individual can undertake for themselves. Others are more a matter of how our society goes about daily life.

First, a word of warning. In all cases, I would exhort any headache sufferer to first get a diagnosis from a fully qualified medical practitioner — more than one, if necessary. There is no protocol that stops you from getting a second opinion or asking for a specialist opinion. It may be that you have had such a diagnosis, and are happy that the medications you are on control your symptoms satisfactorily. You may be reading this book simply to find out more about your condition. In contrast, you may be tired of always taking pills, and feel that they don't help a lot anyway, and you may be reading this book in order to find some treatment strategies to put into practice. But it would be foolhardy to try to treat yourself without first ensuring that the 'migraine' you are suffering from is not in fact a brain tumour.

In addition, recent assessment is important. Just because you have been diagnosed with migraine or stress headaches in the past, it does not mean that you cannot develop a second pathology, such as a stroke or a brain tumour. Any change in the nature, frequency, or severity of your headaches should ring alarm bells.

Throughout this book, I refer to the many factors that relate to the problem of headache. As a doctor who wants to understand the disease process, I am always drawn to scientific data. Sometimes I am able to infect my patients with my enthusiasm. Often, I suspect, they wish I would just get on with the business of finding an answer to their problem. So I have written the book with this in mind. Some people will get all they need from Part II, which focuses on treatment methods — and find themselves reading a much shorter book. But because most people seem to want to know the reasons for their headaches, I did not start with treatments. Many individuals are trying to piece the story together, and learn about the other health implications their headaches have for them and their families. For that reason, I have started by outlining what headaches are, what causes them, and why, giving as much detail as I think I can get away with as I proceed. I do not want any reader to feel intimidated by anatomy and chemistry. Even the very words scare some. So I primarily concentrate on the hard science in Part III.

We all learn in different ways. The way I learn best is to understand the scientific basics first. So if I were a young doctor just starting to go beyond the pharmacotherapy of headache, I would probably start at Chapter 10. If I were a headache sufferer or their friend or family member, I would start at Chapter 1.

I hope the science you meet as you read will help to answer the question every headache sufferer asks at some time: 'Why me?' And I hope that it will give you some new information and strategies when it comes to treating and preventing headaches.

PART I

The Problem of Headache

CHAPTER 1
My Head Hurts: living with headache

'It is astonishing with how little reading a doctor can practise medicine, but it is not astonishing how badly he may do it.'
Sir William Osler

In September 2009, Cindy McCain was a keynote speaker at the 14th Congress of the International Headache Society (IHS) in Philadelphia. IHS is a charity-based organisation for people from all professions who treat headache disorders, and it publishes a respected journal, *Cephalalgia*. McCain, the wife of former presidential candidate John McCain, spoke in the lead-up to the Congress, describing the journey she had travelled since she had first developed migraine (after a hysterectomy at the age of 38). One doctor had described her as neurotic, but she had gone to important events 'throwing up out the car window'. Headaches had caused her to miss a lot of significant events in her children's lives. And it did not take much to set them off — just a sudden drop in barometric pressure (a thunderstorm), odours from cooking, perfume, and wine, or foods such as red meat, chicken, and chocolate.

Then there were the food additives, such as MSG and sulphites. Imagine what such a life would be like if you have a role where you must eat out and deal with people every day.

Among the remedies McCain had tried were acupuncture, acupressure, massage, biofeedback, analgesics, tricyclic antidepressants, and botox. On an island in Micronesia, a medicine man gave her some crushed guava leaves that seemed to help. Either the doctor who called her neurotic was right, or this was one very desperate lady.

And were her headaches a warning sign of other health issues she might face? She had endured a miscarriage and a stroke, unexplained weight loss, and drug addiction. Was she just unlucky, or was some cause-and-effect going on here?

McCain aimed to raise funds to find a satisfactory treatment for migraine. In her attempts to get help, she said, 'I'll do anything, including chew broken glass, if it would help me get rid of this.'[6]

Her treatment journey, the triggers for her headaches, her related health issues, and — not least — her desperate claim that she would be prepared to chew broken glass to fix the problem do, I think, echo the situations and feeling of many migraine and chronic-headache sufferers.

THE EFFECTS OF HEADACHE

If the life of public figures such as McCain requires an imaginative leap, we can look closer to home. You don't have to be a would-be-presidential wife to be affected. In a recent radio report, a headache sufferer, Alison, said: 'As a single parent, it was rather challenging … I remember there were times when I had to get my older son to make dinner for his younger brother, and I was trying to give him instructions as to how to make the lunches, and get friends to come and collect the kids to take them to school because I knew that I couldn't move or I would be sick.'[7]

Alison's neurologist diagnosed migraine. Her story was typical of a migraine sufferer. Headache symptoms vary according to the type of headache, and we will look at some of these categories shortly. Yet even within a category — say, 'tension headache' or 'migraine' — every person will be different.

Of course, pain is the key feature of headache, as demonstrated in the names it is given in various languages. In French, it's *mal à la tête*; in Japanese, *atama ga itai desu*; in Norwegian, *hodepine*; in Catalan, *mal de cap*; in Welsh, *cur pen*; in Italian, *mal di testa*; and of course in English, *headache*. One does not need to be a linguist to get the message; the head is hurting. But headache is more than just pain. Nausea, fatigue, insomnia, loss of confidence, and depression are just some of the symptoms that may accompany it. It can affect your work and your whole life, as the following patients of mine show.

The difficulties of living with headache

It was not hard to give Catherine a label: she was a classic migraineur. Her headaches came regularly each month with her period. She had aura (an uneasy feeling accompanied by visual disturbance), nausea, and vomiting. She had a penchant for chocolate, and because she sometimes got away with eating it, had managed to convince herself that — despite evidence to the contrary — chocolate was not one of the factors in her headaches.

However, Catherine was also a professional classical musician. Time off work was not always an option. Even drugged to the eyeballs with every preventive medicine and treatment you could imagine, she found that her career was in jeopardy.

David was a lawyer in his mid-fifties. He came to me on his wife's insistence that he 'try another approach'. His headaches always began with work stress, and he could feel his jaw clench and his neck stiffen. Sleep could sometimes abort an attack, but if the headache hit, the pain was 'excruciating' and responded poorly to analgesics. Once the headache was established, he would become very nauseous, could not tolerate light, and often ended up vomiting.

Sometimes one headache was followed almost immediately by another. At other times, he could go months without headaches at all. He was a non-smoker on a healthy diet. He could identify no obvious food triggers. He knew that he was sensitive to alcohol and so drank minimally and rarely. David had been to a headache clinic; he had been provisionally diagnosed with cluster headaches. However, it would be easy to make a case for tension headache or cluster headache or migraine. (These classifications are discussed in detail shortly).

Ari was a young builder with a supportive wife, and he had been diagnosed with cluster headaches. He was taking a lot of time off work with headaches he described as 'blinding'. His daily regime of preventive medication was formidable.

He worried about the effects of this on his judgement and balance when up on a roof.

Ari had seen a series of neurologists but favoured his current one, who had prescribed oxygen for the attacks. He found that oxygen had helped him more than anything else. The problem was, what would happen if he was on the roof and needed to grab his oxygen cylinder? What would the welder think when he walked past carrying this thing? Would his boss allow it under occupational health and safety rules? How else could he earn his living without expensive retraining?

Related health issues

People who suffer headaches also have an increased risk of other health problems. Sometimes it is almost impossible to separate cause and effect, but I believe that getting to the bottom of the headache can unlock some of the related issues. They include:

- asthma and sinusitis
- arthritis
- cardiovascular disorders (in older patients)
- chronic fatigue syndrome and multiple chemical sensitivity
- coeliac disease and gluten sensitivity
- complex regional pain syndrome
- inflammatory bowel disease
- insomnia and sleep disorders
- irritable bowel syndrome
- mood disorders (including depression and anxiety)

- neck and spinal pain
- pregnancy sickness
- travel sickness
- vertigo

Asthma and sinusitis

Many patients say that their headaches begin with a sinus infection or a bout of wheezing. Some describe an 'asthma headache'. At least one British study has shown that migraine in children increased the risk of asthma by a factor of 1.59, and that an asthmatic child was 5.5 times more likely to have a parent with migraine than non-asthmatic children. An American headache specialist, Doctor Roger K. Cady, agrees. He believes that asthma (and allergic rhinitis) and headaches (sinus and migraine) are linked. 'Controlling either of those will help the other,' he says.[8]

The immune system of our airways functions to protect us from inhaled toxins. These may be germs and dust, but the chemicals that we will read about (in Chapters 3 and 7) can range from 'irritants' right through to carcinogens. Our reactive airways are trying to protect us from them. Are our headaches trying to do the same thing?

Arthritis

Headache can be a symptom of arthritis in the upper part of the spine. Both rheumatoid arthritis and osteoarthritis can result in pain in the head, generally towards the back but sometimes radiating up to the crown. Sudden withdrawal of arthritis medication can also cause headaches.

Cardiovascular disorders (older patients)

The link here is mainly to stroke in migraine sufferers. This will be discussed in Chapter 5.

Headache sufferers are more likely to have high blood pressure than the general population.[9] Heart and circulatory problems can cause headaches if blood supply to the head is restricted by thickened arteries or clots. In people with a history of heart disease, sudden or severe head pain can be a sign of serious problems and should be evaluated immediately by a doctor. Some drugs prescribed for cardiovascular disease may cause headaches in some people, but these can generally be relieved by altering the medication.

Chronic fatigue syndrome and multiple chemical sensitivity

Professor Martin Pall from Washington State University maintains a website on chemical-free living.[10] A biochemist, he is an expert on the environmental chemicals that affect many people. Headache is a common symptom, and from my perspective, the genetic links to chemical sensitivity are among the most interesting.

In short, a major contributor to chemical sensitivity is the activation of a receptor in our body, the N-methyl-D-aspartate receptor (NMDA receptor). Approximately seven classes of chemical can activate it, and vulnerable people are genetically more sensitive to such effects. For the link to headache pain, see Chapter 5.

The Australian ME/CFS (myalgic encephalomyelitis/chronic fatigue syndrome) Society and the Allergy and Environmental Sensitivity Support and Research Association

(AESSRA) are registered charities that provide valuable resources.[11] Their existence indicates the level of public concern. But despite the increase in complaints from individuals, there is seemingly an even greater increase in potentially suspect products, as instanced by the use of air fresheners in some doctors' surgeries (see Chapter 8).

Many people who suffer from these conditions find that they are affected by their place of work, or by being inside modern buildings with poor ventilation to the outside world. The World Health Organization has found that up to 30 per cent of new and remodelled buildings worldwide may be causing so-called 'sick building syndrome'.[12] This is largely caused by poor indoor air quality, with the presence of moulds and volatile organic compounds.

Coeliac disease and gluten sensitivity

Coeliac disease is a genetically determined autoimmune disease that results in damage to the small intestine whenever gluten is consumed. The symptoms may range from occasional stomach aches through to extreme diarrhoea and weight loss. Not all symptoms relate to the gut, and the neurological system is often targeted. Examples of related conditions include mood disorders, epilepsy, cerebellar ataxia (damage to nerve cells in the part of the brain that controls muscle coordination), premature Alzheimer's, autism, and even some cases of schizophrenia.

Not all people who have coeliac genes develop coeliac disease. Indeed, it is thought that only about one in 20 genetically vulnerable people ever develop clinical coeliac disease. But it seems that once those genes have been switched on (usually in the first few years of life), they are on for life.

Gluten sensitivity has been researched as another risk when the genes are present, although it is also possible in the absence of coeliac genes. As coeliac disease and gluten sensitivity are problems seen increasingly, they are attracting much research interest as prototypes of autoimmune disorders.

Many people, once diagnosed with one of these conditions, have observed that their headaches have abated once they stopped eating gluten. Headache is a common symptom of gluten intolerance of any cause. This subject is discussed further in Chapters 3 and 6.

Complex regional pain syndrome

This is a distressing syndrome whereby pain persists following a relatively minor injury, long after healing is apparently complete. A feature is allodynia: extreme sensitivity to a mild stimulus — such as a light touch, which is experienced as a burning or stinging sensation. We look at allodynia in Chapters 7 and 10.

In very extreme circumstances, this syndrome can lead to atrophy and withering of a limb. Pain clinics see many such patients, and the problem is perplexing.

Recently I saw a patient, herself medically trained, who mentioned that her specialist had commented that the problem ran in families. So we set about looking for the genetic links. Both of us were excited to find that the link was through the NMDA receptors (mentioned above; see also Chapter 13). The chemistry involves an increased release of glutamate, an excitatory chemical central to our discussion of headache.

In 2009, *Cephalalgia* published a study that suggests that

migraineurs, especially those who experience aura, are more at risk of developing this syndrome than people who do not suffer from headaches.[13]

I have three patients with the condition: all of them are migraineurs.

Inflammatory bowel disease

This category includes diseases such as Crohn's, colitis, and ulcerative colitis. Many of these patients experience significant headaches, which are thought to be secondary to a 'leaky gut', meaning that undigested food gets absorbed across the gut lining. Such food particles are normally stopped by 'tight junctions', and the implication for a food link to headache are enormous. In 2013, Doctor Peter H. Green, of Columbia University in New York, conducted a study into coeliac disease and inflammatory bowel disease. He claimed that he expected to see a higher rate of migraines in coeliac patients, but the increased migraine rate he found in the patients with inflammatory bowel disease was a 'complete surprise'.[14]

Insomnia and sleep disorders

Besides the disturbance that the headache itself will bring to sleep, some people, as case studies show, even set alarms to take their medication. Other factors include bruxism (the clenching and grinding of teeth), which is linked to both headache and insomnia. To find the cause is to embark on a chicken-and-egg discussion.

Finally, some interesting research, discussed in Chapter 13, links an adenosine receptor gene that some of us have to both migraine with aura and insomnia.

Irritable bowel syndrome

Although irritable bowel syndrome is a contested term, with doctors disagreeing about what it is and if it exists, it is typically said to involve abdominal pain, bloating, constipation, and/or diarrhoea. Chapter 2 looks at genetic links between headache and irritable bowel syndrome. In Chapter 3, we look some blood tests used in a UK study to assess problematic foods for people with IBS. Some doctors use these same tests in managing patients with headaches. Most migraine sufferers, and many people with headaches of other kinds, comment on a change of bowel habit when they experience a bad headache.

Mood disorders

If your life is dominated by headache, it does not take much imagination to see that you might be prone to problems such as anxiety or depression, or even another serious mental illness. It is obvious that the headache makes you more vulnerable to certain mental conditions such as anxiety, but there are some biochemical links as well. Chapter 2 looks at some 'headache genes' that have been linked to epilepsy, schizophrenia, and anxiety disorders (EAAT2), and a gene linked to alcoholism and depression (SERT). In addition, the MTHFR gene is strongly associated with the autism-spectrum disorders, and is often found in the close relatives of children on this spectrum.

Chapter 3 examines the effect of the various chemicals in our diet, both natural and synthetic, on mood. If we are sensitive to these chemicals, things that we are eating may be responsible both for our mood changes *and* for our headaches.

Even the most conventional doctors often include many nutrients that have a beneficial effect on headache, such as magnesium and the B-group vitamins, in the treatment of mood disorders. If these nutrients are missing from the diet, the concurrence of headache and mood problems should come as no surprise.

A 2008 Israeli study indicated that women who wear too much perfume may do so as the result of a loss of smell, which is linked to depression.[15] This may well be true; however, as Mary's story (Chapter 7) will demonstrate, the reverse may also be true. When we look through the list of toxic effects caused by chemicals, 'headache' and 'central nervous system effects' figure on the list. Central nervous system problems result in both anxiety and depression. And Professor Martin Pall links post-traumatic stress disorder to a constellation of 'unexplained illnesses'; he sees a chemical link in many of these, and the co-morbidity with headache in all of them is well known.[16] The suspect chemicals are further explored in Chapters 7, 12, and 13.

Neck and spinal pain

Many patients with tension headache or migraine report that their headaches begin with tightening of the neck muscles. Researchers have focused on the occipital nerve, which is discussed in Chapter 11. Again, cause and effect are difficult to separate when it comes to links to headaches. Anecdotally, a lot of patients do gain relief for a wide range of headaches from physical therapies such as chiropractic.

Pregnancy sickness

Extreme morning sickness, or *hyperemesis gravidarum*, gained the attention of the press worldwide when it hospitalised the wife of the younger heir to the British throne. Her headache status is unknown to us, but the severe form of this illness has strong links to migraine, as we shall see. The extreme case of Charlotte Brontë was discussed in the introduction, and the link between pregnancy sickness and headaches can also be seen in studies. For instance, a 2001 study found that in a retrospective record review of 37 migraineurs who had gone through pregnancy, 10 (27 per cent) had experienced *hyperemesis gravidarum*.[17]

Travel sickness

Motion sickness, caused by a disturbance in the motion-sensing organs of the inner ear, seems to have some connection with migraine. The symptoms include dizziness, nausea, and vomiting. Many adult migraine sufferers experienced carsickness as children, and migraineurs are five times more likely to suffer motion sickness than the general population. Travel sickness is discussed further in Chapter 4.

Vertigo

Vertigo describes dizziness, in which the individual feels that either they or the environment around them is moving rapidly when in fact everything is stationary, or moving only slightly.

Recently I saw a very distressed young mother who had suffered from severe migraines since puberty and had developed bouts of vertigo after a presumed ear infection.

Her vertigo was so intense that she was not safe to hold her baby. She had seen ear, nose, and throat specialists and neurologists, and had attended a vertigo clinic. The diagnoses she had received included viral labyrinthitis, vestibular neuritis, and Ménière's disease (all of which affect the inner ear), as well as vertiginous migraine. It is not necessary to go into these disorders here, other than to say that vertigo is often a symptom of migraine, and migraineurs seem to be more at risk of these other conditions, which her doctors had considered. Currently she is being tested for various 'headache genes' (Chapter 2), in the hope that appropriate support nutrients will help her to regain some level of normality.

It is my guess that she will be much better managed if we can reduce the amount of glutamate in her diet — especially as MSG, but also that which occurs naturally in any food. This would be my advice to any headache sufferer, or anyone with significant vertiginous symptoms. Glutamate is extensively discussed throughout this book.

Effects on work

The problems of headache are not confined to the pain of an attack, as we have just seen. There is the anxiety of wondering when it will next strike. And if you are anxious at work, can you do your best?

Many people with headache suffer insomnia. If you are having two or three headaches a week, when do you catch up on that sleep? What if you are a truck driver: are you safe to be in control of a vehicle? Maybe the cause of your insomnia is dietary; the same foods that trigger headaches may also trigger insomnia. Maybe you have trouble sleeping because you wake during the night in order to take preventive medications. But a vicious cycle can develop: headaches beget insomnia, insomnia begets headache. A sleep-deprived worker is not a productive worker.

Those with headaches who also get irritable bowel syndrome may try to avoid MSG, but what's in the food from the cafeteria or the take-away shop near their office? Should they get up half an hour earlier to make a 'safe' lunch?

Do occupational hazards, besides stress, *contribute* to the headaches? Train drivers may experience a strobe effect as they alternate through tunnels and bright light. Office workers might be subjected to flickering fluorescent lights or pungent air freshener in the washrooms. Are these chemicals increasing the risk not only of headache, but also of chronic fatigue syndrome and multiple chemical sensitivity? The headaches are not the *cause* of these problems; rather, the environmental factors that trigger headaches may be causing other problems as well.

In short, the workplace may offer serious challenges to the headache sufferer, and the sufferer may in turn be at risk in the workplace. Whether they are professionals, such as Catherine and David; skilled tradespeople, such as Ari; single mothers, such as Alison; or truck drivers, teachers, or factory workers, headache sufferers all face difficulties in getting on with their jobs and their lives.

Effects on family, friends, and colleagues

The effects of headaches are not confined to the individual. Alison, as we saw, had to get friends to take her kids to school. Her older son was cooking for his brother, so you have to wonder how his needs were met when she was sick. Catherine is single and has few close relatives. Her sister worries about her and adds her to the people she feels responsible for, along with her young children. David's firm accommodates his time away from work, but clients with court attendances need David in person. The practice principals are concerned to do the right thing by him, but they need to keep the business viable. His wife feels that their weekends are spent with David asleep or doing catch-up work. Ari and his wife want to start a family, but both are worried about how they will pay the mortgage if his job is in doubt.

That's the problem with headache. When you are well, you are well. You don't want to take early retirement or retrain. But you just don't know what's going to happen next, and the people around you can't make plans.

CLASSIFICATION OF HEADACHES

The introduction put forward the idea that headaches can be classified as primary or secondary. Secondary headaches are those that result from specific pathology, such as sinusitis or concussion, and their management should focus on the underlying cause.

The International Headache Society has undertaken the mammoth task of classifying primary headaches. The result is hardly simple (even the convenors of the society admit that it is too complex for them to commit to memory!), but does have its uses. However, knowing the classification system is just that — an exercise in taxonomy.

Doctors like to classify headaches because then they can follow treatment guidelines. Many patients I see have a clear idea of what kind of headache they have — say, typical migraine, or pure tension headache. Others are less certain. Here is a list of names that doctors use. However, if you feel you do not neatly fit one of these categories, you are not alone.

- **Atypical facial pain** (trigeminal autonomic cephalalgias). This is a name for a group of headaches, generally marked by intense, short bursts of head or neck pain.
- **Chronic daily headache.** This is a classification for headaches that don't fit neatly into another category. Any of the headaches in this list can morph into this condition, which is as it sounds: a head pain every, or almost every, day.
- **Cluster headache.** This resembles migraine, but the pain is so intense that it is often referred to as 'the suicide headache'. The headaches tend to occur in groups, or clusters, hence the name.
- **Medication overuse headache.** This type of headache, caused by an over-reliance on pain medication, has close links to chronic daily headache.
- **Migraine.** Key features of migraine are pain, typically on one side of the head, and vomiting. It may occur with aura (MA) or without aura (MO); the latter is known as 'common migraine'.
- **Paroxysmal hemicrania.** This is an intense headache, with severe pain on one side of the head, often

accompanied by a weeping eye and swelling eyelid on that side. It is frequently confused with migraine.
- **Tension headache.** This is the most common type of headache, and can be divided into three subsets: *tension-type headache*, *episodic tension-type headache*, and *chronic tension-type headache*.

This is a brief summary of the main headache classifications. A fuller discussion occurs in Chapter 10.

The diagnostic dilemma

When a patient gives me a 'classic' history, diagnosis can be straightforward. If someone gets headaches with aura, vomiting, and visual disturbance, it is not hard to call them migraines. But often it is difficult to squeeze the story into any of the forms listed above, or sometimes even to discern a pattern at all. The most we can say is that any descriptors give us a framework in which we can think about headache. Genetic studies now lend support to the idea of specific pathologies in each and every case of headache.

The risk is that when we start to use a Chinese-menu approach to diagnosis, we inevitably oversimplify. If I decide to sort out my bookshelves, do I sort the books by size or by subject matter, by author, or by some other criterion, and what do I do with the books that belong in more than one category? Headaches may be sorted by underlying pathology, genetic basis, response to medication, clinical presentation, and so on. The selection criteria may cloud the purpose of the exercise.

Perhaps another way of thinking about headaches could go like this.

When we experience pain or discomfort, it's reasonable to assume that the body is trying to tell us something. That 'something' may be as simple as needing to move away from the fire because we're too hot, or to stop standing on a piece of broken glass. That is the purpose of pain. The 'message' is important because it guides corrective action. But what if the message is out of all proportion to the threat?

My thinking is that some event in our internal or nearby environment kick-starts a conversation between one part of the body and another, one neurotransmitter and another, one hormone and another. But just as a conversation can become an argument, or peace talks can end in war, a neural or hormonal message can turn into something more threatening. Many factors contribute, and there is no one Factor X. If we continue the analogy, war erupts when there is an interplay among a multitude of contributing factors. An isolated headache may serve the purpose of sending us to bed when we are overtired or stressed, but often headaches come like a bolt from the blue. What can be the purpose of making us miss our best friend's wedding or our son's graduation?

In any case, tight classification systems may result in deterministic thinking and semantic determinism. When we classify illnesses by name, we are tempted to assume a single cause, and even to assume that the name somehow explains the disease. And, of course, there is a whole pharmaceutical industry just waiting to find the drug that controls the disease that has that name. There is big money in that, since headache affects more than one in ten of us. Let us say that you get migraine because you have migraine genes, and that I suffer from 'tension headaches' and so my headaches must be caused by stress. Thus you are prescribed the latest migraine drug, while I get a psychotropic medication to manage my stress levels.

But this oversimplifies the problem and may leave out other important factors. What if both of us have a gene that makes us intolerant of sulphite additives? (After all, 20 per cent of us do; see Chapter 10.) When we get a load of additives through our food — as is easy in the modern supermarket diet — we may not sleep well, and the next day we will not handle the stress of our jobs. We end up with a 'migraine', or 'tension headaches'. Perhaps we should re-evaluate our diets and get rid of the additives, rather than taking the latest medication for our symptoms.

Someone else may have a dental malalignment, or grind his teeth and clench his jaw in response to stress. By a feedback loop through the sympathetic nervous system, he develops tension headaches that would be best managed with a dental brace or meditation.

Someone who has 'tension headaches' may also have one of the well-known 'migraine genes' (Chapter 2) and sometimes experience classic migraine. Does the tendency to tension headache interact with the migraine predisposition independently, or are the biochemical determinants of one headache likely to feed into the other? The current medical approach to headache, in its minimalist form, is to take a history, classify the headache, and prescribe medication appropriate for that type of headache. The more thorough doctor might add a full physical examination, appropriate blood tests, referral to a specialist, and lifestyle advice.

Of course the latter is the better medical practice. But the lives of the Cindy McCains of this world, no doubt in receipt of expert medical care, remain limited by headaches. So what is missing?

From the waiting room to the doctor's chair

It was Friday morning and I arrived early at work. Marjorie was not normally my patient — this was some time ago, and I was new to that practice.— but she was sitting in the waiting room dry-retching into the bucket between her knees. Her husband sat beside her, looking drawn. This had been going on since the early hours of the morning. The doctor who normally saw her was up in Maternity delivering a baby. The other patients in the waiting room looked disconcerted, to say the least, so I took her into my office and got out her file.

Marjorie had been diagnosed by a specialist with frequent episodes of classic migraine. There was a family history because her mother and her aunt were both migraine sufferers. She was not keen on daily prevention tablets because they had side-effects and she felt that they made little difference. She had originally relied on ergot-based (amine) tablets when the attacks began — today, triptans would probably have been prescribed. She had noticed that when she got a lot of headaches, she seemed to develop a dependence on the tablets. It was as if the more headaches she got and the more she tried to treat them, the more headaches she was going to get.

Although not all presentations are as dramatic as Marjorie's, on any day of the week at least one patient in my waiting room will have come to see me about chronic headache. The waiting rooms of GPs in any Western country will contain such patients, looking for prescriptions, certificates for work, and sometimes referral to specialists.

Although 'tension' has been identified as the most common type of headache, most of these patients do not identify themselves as having tension headaches. Maybe this is because the typical person with tension headaches only has them occasionally, and just puts up with them when they occur. Maybe they simply don't know what to call their headaches.

Because of my interest in this area, I tend to see the people whose lives are ruled by headaches. They are the ones who turn down the invitation to be their best friend's bridesmaid or refuse a promotion because they can't count on being well. Many of them tell me that they get 'migraines', but others assume that they cannot have migraine because they have never had an aura or seen flashing lights. Some of them say that pills don't work. Others have been to headache clinics and found pills that work but have unpleasant side effects, or provide only temporary relief. Over the years, I have felt a tension between the desire to get the right diagnosis and the competing desire not to classify chronic problems into neat little boxes.

Not long ago, I was admitted to hospital for a simple day procedure that required an overnight fast beforehand. The woman in the bed opposite me was in for a similar procedure, but there was concern as to whether it could go ahead. She had woken that morning with a headache that had gradually developed into a full-blown migraine. It seemed to me that the probable precipitant was the lack of her bedtime pot of tea and her standard pot of morning coffee. (She mentioned these when asked if she had observed the instruction to take 'nil by mouth'.) I did not like to ask whether she used these drinks to wash down regular migraine-prevention pills, but I wondered whether she was undergoing a double withdrawal.

The severe headache that sometimes accompanies gastroenteritis is often attributed to dehydration caused by vomiting. Any vomiting that accompanies severe head pain should alert the doctor to the possibility of a cerebral event. But more often, the gastroenteritis headache is caused by caffeine withdrawal, as the patient goes without their regular fix.

The woman in the bed near me was not my patient, and all I could do was wonder about her story. But with the patient sitting opposite me in my office, I have a responsibility, and I need an approach that will work for both of us.

Firstly, I need to satisfy myself that there has been adequate investigation to rule out 'nasties', such as tumour or aneurysm. This might be based on the headache history and a physical examination, and may also include a CT scan or an MRI. Recent assessment by a specialist neurologist is always reassuring. Then I ask the patient about their life, occupation, family, personal relationships, and so on. I need to know the context of their headaches, and this can give me the clues I need in order to work out the causes and the management of their problem. Family history of headache and other illnesses is important. Important too is the story of how the headaches present, what has been tried, what has worked, what the patient suspects precipitates the headaches, and so on.

With this information, I start to form some hypotheses about what is going on. At this stage they can only be theories;

maybe that is all they can ever be, because absolute proof is elusive in medicine, in science, and in life in general. However, with some hypothesis about the causation, I can hope to make a difference. And I begin by helping the patient to take ownership of the headache.

The analogy of a loaded gun

I try to fit what I have heard into a framework that the patient can connect to, using the analogy of a loaded gun. Like all analogies, it has both uses and limitations.

Think about it like this: some of us are born with the headache 'gun', while others are not. Such an analogy can be used for other illnesses, such as asthma, depression, coeliac disease, or even obesity, but let us stick with headaches right now. The 'gun' is the many genetic factors that make us vulnerable to headache of one sort or another. We will see shortly how much is known about the genes for various types of headache. If you don't have the genes, you probably won't get the headaches. Some people get more than their fair share of headache genes, and others are blessed by seeming to get none at all.

The next step is to imagine what puts the bullets, which I think of as common foods, in the gun. Is it certain food additives or chemicals?

The third step is to find the factors that either pull the trigger or protect the gun from becoming 'trigger happy'. In this last case, I'm thinking in terms of locks on the trigger. The patient may have already answered some of these questions for me; in other cases, we need to work them out.

This analogy is simplistic. But I think that more things

are missed in scientific endeavour and medical research because they are too obvious than because they are too difficult.

So if we return to Marjorie, and look at the stories of some other patients as well, maybe we can see how the 'gun, bullets, and triggers' approach might apply.

My guess was that Marjorie had developed ergot-withdrawal headaches (we shall read more about this in Chapter 9). Many attacks began in the early hours of the morning, and rapidly led to nausea and vomiting. It was a balancing act to get in with treatment before she was unable to keep the pills down — and to counter her desire not to take anything unless she really needed it. Marjorie had not yet developed the habit of setting the alarm for 4 a.m. to pre-empt her symptoms, as other patients have done, noting, 'Once the headache wakes you, doctor, it's already too late.'

We knew little of the genetics of migraine (with the possible exception of familial hemiplegic migraine) in the early 1990s, but it was reasonable to assume that she had the migraine 'gun'. There was a family history, and the migraines followed a 'classic' pattern. Although I was in the habit of putting patients on elimination diets, that morning was clearly not the time for such a discussion. From the desperate look in Marjorie's eyes, it was obvious that anything other than symptomatic relief would be irrelevant. I gave her a shot of pethidine and another injection for vomiting, and sent her home to sleep it off. As she was leaving, I remarked that if she wanted to see me some time when she felt well, we could perhaps discuss a different strategy.

I was surprised when she returned some time later. I explained my analogy of a loaded gun, bullets, and triggers: that common foods can act as bullets and a variety of things can act as triggers. We went through the elaborate steps involved in an elimination diet. Marjorie certainly looked dubious as I ruled out most of her favourite foods, telling me, 'But I've been eating that all my life.' But she was willing to give it a go. Chapters 3 and 6 discuss in detail the rationale, types, and protocols of elimination diets, but to explain broadly, you stick to a list of 'safe' foods for about four to six weeks. If the headaches disappear, foods are reintroduced one at a time, and ideally the culprit foods will become apparent.

I did not see Marjorie again for several months, and then one day she came running after me in the street. 'You won't believe me, doctor,' she said. 'It was the green food colouring.' At first it took me a moment to place her, but when I did, I realised that, having done the diet, she had found that the principal thing that provoked her headache was food colouring. It turned out that she had been in the habit of drinking large quantities of a low-calorie green cordial.

From my point of view, this made sense. There was no doubt that Marjorie was a victim of classic migraine. She had a family history, and something she was doing was loading the gun for her. What seemed to be triggering the attacks was the overnight 'withdrawal' effect of going only a few hours without the medication. In summary, she clearly had the headache 'gun'. There was no single Factor X: her genetic makeup, at least one food additive, and medication (over)use were all involved. The removal of the green food-colouring 'bullet' helped to unload the gun, and as it did so, she was able to break the dependence on medication. With no issues of medication dependence, she had broken the whole cycle. She was able to become free of both headaches and drugs, with ownership of the solution in her hands. I have to say that it is rarely as easy as this, but that woman's life was transformed by the removal of a single food additive.

Since then I have had another patient whose worst migraines were triggered by Midori, a bright-green alcoholic drink. She had many other food triggers, but green dye was quite outstanding in its effect. I have been unable, either by internet search or by reading the label, to find out what the colouring used in Midori might be. Possibly this is because of an Australian grandfathering clause that allows imported or longstanding products to contain ingredients without labelling them. However, a bottle of crème de menthe and another similar product both acknowledged the use of E102 (tartrazine, a yellow food colouring) and E133 (brilliant blue) in producing a bright-green liqueur. Interestingly, green is one of the food colours now under severe restriction in the United Kingdom, since a 2007 study addressing hyperactivity in children.[18]

We turn now to another patient, seen more recently, in whom the guns, bullets, and triggers are different, but where the same approach gave a good outcome.

John's story
John worked from home. He had previously had a good job as an accountant with a big firm, but although everyone was initially prepared to accommodate his frequent sick days, he had become uncomfortable when other staff made comments

about his absences. He knew he pulled his weight by taking work home, and on the days he felt well, he would come in early and go home late to make up his hours. All up, he was probably working longer hours than most.

It would be easy to make assumptions about 'obsessive accountants', but as I got to know him, I learned to enjoy his wry sense of humour and to admire his determination not to let headaches ruin his life. As part of this, he had become a freelance worker, so that he was able to adjust his workload around the headaches.

John had an impressive array of medications from a headache clinic. He took these daily in divided treatments, and also kept them beside his bed. He had developed a habit of taking them on waking — a remnant from the days when he worked in an office, because failure to do so had usually resulted in an early morning headache.

John did not wear aftershave, and his house was low in chemicals. He already knew that he had a bad response to perfumes and aerosol sprays, and avoided them. We talked about stress, teeth grinding, and other matters.

Then we went through the dietary factors and discussed an elimination diet. But for John, the big thing was coffee. He drank a lot of it, with milk. Life without coffee or milk seemed to be unthinkable.

The removal of caffeinated drinks and all dairy products is essential to the elimination diet. Quite dreadful headaches can occur in the initial phase of such a trial because of caffeine withdrawal. John was not keen to go there. I suggested that we do a staged removal. He was to switch to black coffee — because I suspected that milk was acting as an important 'bullet' — and also gradually lower his caffeine intake.

Without dairy products and with a gradual reduction in caffeine, John's headaches soon reduced dramatically. He also began taking magnesium tablets.

I see John's outcome as a partial success; he could not get the coffee down to less than four or five cups a day, but the improvement in his headaches did make it possible to reduce his medication. Dependence on medication had certainly compounded his problems, and was undoubtedly linked to the caffeine dependence. In turn, overnight withdrawal was what had led to the early morning headaches.

When I last saw John, he had managed to wean off regular medications and was now using pills only when headaches threatened. They, in turn, responded to medication much more readily. He continued to drink black coffee at the reduced dose, but was headache-free most days. It was a solution he could live with.

CHAPTER 2
The Gun: why headache can run in families

'Mortals are but playthings of the gods ...'
OEDIPUS REX

Imagine that you have come to see me as a patient to discuss your headaches. You have not been to my practice before, so you have been asked to come half an hour before your scheduled appointment time. After my receptionist has taken your details, you go into the procedures room, where the practice nurse takes a finger-prick blood sample. When I call you in, you begin by telling me some things about your history, and that your main concern is headache.

After a while, I open up the file we have made on you and click on a tab marked 'genetic profile'. We have this as a result of the blood test my nurse did just a few minutes ago. Together we study the screen, and I walk you through the different gene variants that increase your susceptibility to headache. You seem to have some genes pointing towards 'migraine'. Are they genes for common, or 'classic', migraine, or is there a suggestion of cluster headaches and tension headaches as well?

I also look at your HLA haplotype. This is a blood group found on the white cells in the blood that, among other things, will tell me something of your racial background and to what foods you are likely to be intolerant. It may even be the basis for finding you a donor, should you ever need a kidney transplant.

This scenario sounds far-fetched. We already understand the science, but the technology for fast, cheap profiling like this is not yet available. And we are only in the early days of our understanding: we do not know which genes track to which diagnosis, or which *combinations* of genes cause problems, especially in their interactions with one another. There are other issues to take into account as our knowledge of epigenetics grows. 'Epigenetics' is a term for chemical changes in specific genes, or in the proteins they produce, which control how the information in the genes is used. (For more, see Chapters 12 and 13.)

In the lifetime of many of us, such analyses will be possible, or even routine. They will apply not only to headaches, but also to everything from arthritis to cancer, osteoporosis to diabetes. No health issue will go uncharted.

WHAT WE KNOW ABOUT GENETICS AND HEADACHES

As increasing access to genetic information reveals a multitude of 'headache genes', it might seem that the many people who get headaches are just victims of a malevolent genome. But as we look at the genetics, I think we can begin to see things from another angle.

When we can identify all of the genes in a headache sufferer, we will be able to show that many of us bear several of these culprit genes. Is this just chance, or is it bad design? I doubt it's the latter. I think we will find that those genes are normally there to serve some other purpose, and they only give us headaches when we thwart their real function. To put it another way, these genes have existed in the human genome for many thousands of years, probably with minimal impact.

Are headaches mentioned frequently or only rarely in ancient literature, such as the Bible? This is a question for the medical anthropologist rather than the modern family doctor, but I suspect that in ancient times headaches cast a much shorter shadow than they do today.

When it comes to headaches, what can genetics tell us now?

What follows is solid reading. If you skip this chapter, you can still follow the discussion in this book, but for the curious, some genetic background will remove the mystery surrounding headaches. And it will certainly help to answer the question 'Why me?'

The genetics is exciting because it reveals that simple vitamin and mineral supplements may reduce headaches for many people, or even get rid of the problem for them entirely. We will look at some of these supplements as we go.

Polymorphism and SNiPs

Before we embark on our discussion of genetics, you need to know that most genes may occur in several versions, which are called 'variants' or 'alleles'. A gene that has several versions is said to be 'polymorphic'. The genes for skin and hair colour are good examples of polymorphic genes.

Usually when a gene varies from the normal or most common form(s), the change is minor, and is referred to as a 'single nucleotide polymorphism', or SNP. This is pronounced 'snip' when spoken, and for ease of reading, in this book we will write it as SNiP. Sometimes you will see the word 'mutation', meaning a SNiP. 'Mutation' is used for rare variations, usually in the context of serious conditions. The distinction is linguistic as much as anything else.

It is hard to accept that anyone ever got a headache as a result of a deficiency of aspirin, triptan, or paracetamol. In the account of Cindy McCain in Chapter 1, it is clear that she was poorly served by the system. Her miscarriage and stroke are pointers to a SNiP in a particular gene — MTHFR, which we will discuss shortly. When she had her children, not much was known about this gene, but by the time she gave her dramatic story to the International Headache Society in 2009, we knew a lot. Our knowledge raises several questions. Has she been prescribed B vitamins, and, if not, what are her future risks of stroke? Does she still use cosmetics? (See Chapter 7.) Despite seeing what are no doubt the best available headache specialists, she still relies on a 'daily regimen of pills'.

Some of us seem to be *genetically wired* to have an exaggerated pain response. But there are simple and safe things that even these extra-sensitive people can try for their headaches.

HEADACHE GENES

Let us look at the research into 'headache genes'. Until now, such testing has been expensive, and it has been difficult to find out which of these genes you have. Recently, this has all changed, through the introduction of an online service known as 23andMe, which I am using in an increasing number of cases. (It is under challenge at present by the US Food and Drug Administration, and I worry that the motivation for the challenge may be spurious. For more on this test, see Appendix 2.)

As your doctor, I might try to infer what your genetic influences might be, or do some other tests that are readily available, to guess at the diagnosis. Or I might back several horses at once — especially as most of the treatments are simple and inexpensive. For more about treatments, see Chapters 8 and 9, and for a fuller description of the clinical picture of types of headache, see Chapter 10.

Genes associated with migraine with aura (MA)

The genetic work done in association with migraine has focused on two key areas: blood flow and hormones.

- The genes relating to blood flow have long names, which are abbreviated to MTHFR, MTRR, and ACE D.
- The genes for hormonal influences are known as ESR1 and PGR.

Before we go into detail about these two groups of genes, let's just note that people who have the particular genes for either vascular or hormonal variations are 8.6 times more likely to suffer migraine than those who have a no-risk genetic profile. These variables are subject to ongoing study.[19]

MTHFR: a gene helped by folic acid

MTHFR is a well-researched headache gene, and exciting findings point towards remarkably simple solutions for the people who have certain SNiPs in this gene.

We all have a gene for MTHFR. In fact, we have two, one from Mum and one from Dad. The question is whether we have a SNiP in one of those genes that makes us at greater risk of migraine. Perhaps we have a SNiP in *both* of them: what is called being 'homozygous' for the problem.

The gene is located on chromosome 1 and tells our body to make an enzyme called MTHFR, or methylene tetrahydrofolate reductase. If I rattle this name off in a lecture, it usually draws a laugh — even when the audience is a group of doctors. It seems to be about as meaningful as if I had used the name of a Welsh railway station. But it is a fascinating gene, and two of its SNiPs are linked to problems from headaches through to infertility.

What does this gene do?

Put simply, it helps determine the manner in which we handle folic acid (also called folate). The 'wild' or most robust versions of the gene are known for having a 677C and 1298A conformation. This is because there are known potential trouble spots at two locations, called 677 and 1298, on the gene. The variants, 677C>T and 1298A>C, have been linked to a range of problems, including migraine and post-menopausal stroke. There is an increased risk of cardiovascular disease in any individual who carries them.

These days, most people are aware of the various uses of folic acid. For example, we advise a woman planning a pregnancy to take folic acid supplements to reduce her risk of having a baby with spina bifida. The long-running Nurses Health Study showed that women who took folic acid supplements reduced their risk of bowel cancer.[20] Participants who drank alcohol had an increased risk of breast cancer, but if they also took folic acid supplements, their risk was the same as the non-drinkers'.

Another key role of folic acid is to aid in a chemical process called methylation. Methylation is such an important reaction in biology that life would not function without it. Some are poor methylators, and these people are prone to headaches — among other health problems. (Other 'methylating' factors include SAMe, and vitamins B6 and B12. See Diagram 1 and Chapter 10.)

So let us return to the migraine research. Recent studies have indicated that those with the 'faulty' MTHFR variant, 677C>T, accumulate more homocysteine than other people because of reduced methylation. Homocysteine is an amino acid we make in our body. To make it, our bodies use another amino acid, methionine, which comes from food. But when methionine gives up its methyl group to 'methylate' something, it becomes homocysteine. High levels of homocysteine are known to be toxic. The homocysteine needs to be turned back into methionine by getting another methyl group from folic acid.

The variants in the MTHFR gene represent a partial roadblock in this process of converting homocysteine back to

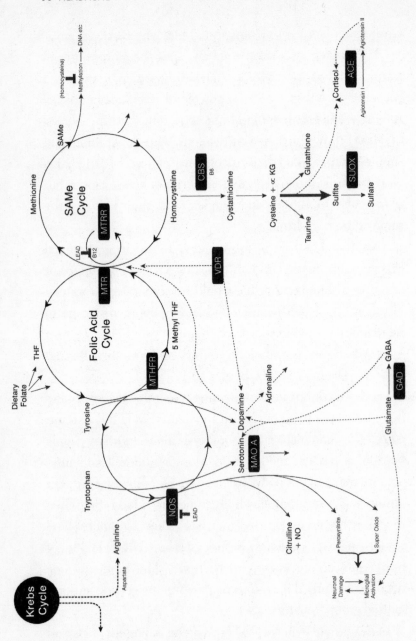

Diagram 1: Methylation cycle

methionine. High levels of homocysteine are an important suspect when it comes to migraine. If the person has two copies of the 'faulty' gene, things can be even worse.

What has the research found so far?

In 2009, Professor Lyn Griffiths and her team from the Genomics Research Centre at Griffith University published a study. The centre is part of a genome-wide association study that was established by the National Institute of Health — with international contributors sharing information — to look at disease profiles on people and at certain 'suspect' SNiPs.[21] The study showed that all migraineurs, whether they carried no, one, or two copies of the 677C>T variant, lowered their homocysteine levels when they took supplements of vitamin B6, B12, and folic acid. Those with two copies of the 'faulty' variant lowered their homocysteine levels the least. Those with no or one copy of the variant improved significantly when taking these supplements, as rated on the Migraine Disability Assessment Test (known as MIDAS). Those with two copies of the faulty gene did not reduce their migraine disability rating at these doses of supplementation. Further trials are underway to see if those with two copies of the faulty gene may respond to higher doses of the supplementation.

Another approach to reducing homocysteine would be to use a more active form of folic acid, known as 5-MTHF, and this is my preferred option. Still other doctors use a form of folic acid known as 'folinic acid'. These options are discussed further in Chapter 8.

So this link with folic acid and accumulation of homocysteine relates to two particular SNiPs in the MTHFR gene.

To complicate things, a gene can have more than one SNiP, meaning that an individual may have problems at both sites. The 1298A>C variant appears to be especially problematic for female migraineurs.

Can I be tested to see if I have a SNiP in this gene?

Yes, most laboratories test for 677C>T and 1298A>C. You may have to pay privately for it, and it can be at a reasonable cost. For further information, see Appendix 2.

How do these SNiPs lead to headache and pain?

If we look at Diagram 1, we see how the poor methylation that can result from these MTHFR variants may mean that folic acid cannot be utilised properly. The results of this include:

- increases in homocysteine
- altered production of neurotransmitters, such as dopamine and serotonin[22]
- reduced repair of damaged gut tissue or leaky gut
- problems with myelination of nerves.[23]

In addition to this, any adverse effect, over the left-hand side of the diagram, caused by poor methylation, may make the person more susceptible to glutamate, the excitatory neurotransmitter associated with pain and neuronal damage.

The significance of these factors will become apparent as we discuss chronic headache and problems that go with it.

MTRR: a gene helped by folic acid and B12

A gene found on chromosome 5 is responsible for the production of methionine synthase reductase, or MTRR.

This is another enzyme involved in methylation, and it needs supplies of both vitamin B12 and folic acid. It supports yet another enzyme, MTR, in turning homocysteine back to methionine (see Diagram 1). The Genomics Research Centre study found that carriers of a variant known as MTRR 66G were overrepresented among female migraineurs. A female who had not only this MTRR 66G variant but also the relevant MTHFR 1298 variant faced a five-fold increase in her risk of migraine.

Another factor that feeds into the mix is lead exposure, which can intensify the problems. So that explodes any simplistic account of the 'genetic' or 'lifestyle' aspect of modern-day headaches. We have inherited these unfortunate genes from our forebears. But because their diets were fresh and full of B12 and folic acid, and there was not such a predominance of lead-based paints or petrol to challenge them, they probably never knew about their genetic tendency to headaches.

ACE D: a gene made worse by a high-salt diet

The acronym ACE stands for angiotensin-1 converting enzyme. The enzyme plays a role in regulating blood pressure and electrolyte balance. An association has been found between migraine and the D variant of this gene, especially if it is accompanied by the MTHFR variant C677T (aka 677C>T).[24] Let us imagine how this particular gene might work, both for us and against us, in its control of our body's fluid balance.

The ACE gene is concerned with the body's management of sodium and potassium, which is called the electrolyte balance. We need both of these minerals, and in the correct ratio. If the diet contains less than the ideal amount of each, the body tries to do the balancing act for us. In particular, the kidneys attempt to sort things out so that we remain in balance.

However, our genetic makeup also has a role to play. Some people are 'salt retainers', who respond rapidly to a high salt load with fluid retention, swollen ankles, and even high blood pressure. We might wonder what is going on here. How could this possibly be advantageous? But if you think about it, tribal people who had to make long desert treks in hot weather would have benefitted from a genetic tendency to retain salt and fluid, losing less precious sodium through sweat and resisting dehydration. A similar benefit would have been found in the tropics, where diarrhoeal disease was a common cause of death, due to loss of water and electrolytes. Retaining salt and fluid might keep you alive.

Compare this with the situation in the 21st century. In the salt-laden diet based on products found in the modern supermarket, there are five or more units of sodium to every unit of potassium. By contrast, in a primitive diet the ratio was completely reversed, at about one unit of sodium, or even less, to five of potassium. And of course that means an overall 25-fold variation. Our ancestors consumed much less sodium and much more potassium. One way to redress the imbalance is to increase our potassium intake by consuming more fresh fruit and vegetables. People who live on salty snacks and don't eat a lot of fruit and vegetables have the double whammy of extra sodium and very little potassium. If you have a gene that favours the retention of salt, and at least one of the genes linked to migraine is affected by salt, the question might become not what is the best *drug* to treat your headaches, but what is the best *diet*.

ESR1: a gene that helps us understand 'hormonal' headaches

Now we have looked at the genes relating to blood flow, we turn to the genes that affect hormones. The ESR1 gene, found on chromosome 6, codes for an oestrogen receptor. At this point, research seems to support the hypothesis that a variant called G594A is linked to migraines.[25]

Women have more oestrogen, and more oestrogen receptors, than men, so the impact of the ESR1 gene may be one reason why women are more prone to migraine than men. The connection also helps explain the cyclical nature of women's migraines.

Worryingly, the ESR1 gene has also been linked by Doctor Amanda Shearman and others to an increased risk of stroke, especially in post-menopausal female migraineurs.[26] The link between stroke and migraine may be explained by platelets, the white blood cells that make our blood sticky. Platelets can clump together and cause clots. Strokes caused by clots are called thrombotic strokes. (Another cause of strokes is bleeding, in which case they are called haemorrhagic strokes.) Small clots are behind some 'mini-strokes' (see Chapter 5). Extra oestrogen, in birth-control pills or hormone replacement therapy, can cause thrombotic strokes.

How might we reduce that risk? Most Western women these days have taken a hormonal contraceptive or had hormone replacement therapy. Women with headaches may studiously avoid these medications *because* of their headaches, and still feel that their hormones are against them. Our bodies produce hormones, and in addition, the world around us is full of environmental 'hormones'. Both plastics (petro-chemicals) and pesticides degrade to oestrogenic molecules, often referred to as 'gender benders' or 'hormone disrupters'. A more accurate term would be 'xeno-oestrogen', often wrongly confused with natural plant 'oestrogens' such as soy, whose correct designation is 'phyto-oestrogen'.

Bisphenol A (BPA) has oestrogenic effects and is banned in some countries; unfortunately, Australia, the United Kingdom, and the United States are not among them. The woman who drinks water or soft drink from the average plastic bottle is exposing herself to a variety of oestrogenic molecules. Then there is the whole range of cosmetic and beauty products, further discussed in Chapter 7. All of these react with a woman's oestrogen receptors.

PGR: another hormone gene

Another gene connected with hormones is the progesterone receptor gene (PGR) on chromosome 1. One variant of this gene, known as the PROGINS variant, has been shown to have some association with migraine in women.[27] Present in up to 30 per cent of the population, it has also been studied in connection with breast and ovarian cancer.

Sensitivity to progesterone may help explain the relationship between pregnancy and migraine. Some women not normally bothered with migraine develop problems when they become pregnant. Others lose their migraines when pregnant, and the reason awaits elucidation. Other factors besides progesterone levels may be at work in these people. Magnesium is important in hormone function, and supplements are worth a try.

TRESK: a breakthrough gene?

The UK's Migraine Action group hailed 26 September 2010, the day the discovery of the gene KCNK 18 was announced, as a red-letter day. Doctor Zameel Cader, a researcher from the University of Oxford, called it a 'once-in-a-generation find'.[28]

The researchers looked at people who had migraine with aura, but excluded those who had symptoms of familial hemiplegic migraine (discussed shortly). They found that a gene located on chromosome 10, KCNK 18, is reponsible for the production of a protein called TRESK. In its normal state, this protein controls the electrical activity (excitability) of certain nerve cells in the trigeminal ganglia and the dorsal root ganglia. These are structures known to be part of the pain pathways in migraine, and are discussed in Chapter 11. The authors describe KCNK 18 as a 'potassium channel gene', and a mutated form has been linked to pain control in migraine.

Yet the excitement surrounding the discovery of the TRESK gene seemed to fade in the ensuing weeks. My feeling is that it will probably turn out to be a just another piece in a very complex puzzle.

Genes associated with common migraine (MO)

Now that we have surveyed the genes that are implicated in migraine with aura, we turn to the genetic aspects of common migraine. The knowledge that is emerging prompts the question: does MSG make you sick?

EAAT2: a gene linking migraine to irritable bowel syndrome

In August 2010, the international consortium GWAS announced that they had discovered a gene for common migraine on chromosome 11.[29] This gene controls a protein called EAAT2, or excitatory amino-acid transporter type 2. EAAT2 is responsible for clearing glutamate from nerve synapses in the brain (and gut). Some versions of the gene are less effective than others in doing this job.

The term 'glutamate' is often used interchangeably with 'glutamic acid'. It is an important molecule in human chemistry, and among other things it acts as a neurotransmitter. Glutamate occurs naturally in the food chain. One of its functions is to send signals to the brain to 'produce pain'.

No discussion on headaches can progress far before glutamate becomes involved. One reason for this is the widespread addition of MSG, a direct source of dietary glutamate, to our food. If you have a high intake of glutamate in your food (more on this in Chapters 3 and 6), you need plenty of the EAAT2 protein to remove it.

During a migraine attack, glutamate is released in the brain. This, along with the release of potassium ions, is the last step in what is referred to as the 'migraine cascade', the events leading up to a migraine attack. Although the research on EAAT2 does not specifically demonstrate *sensitivity* to MSG in common migraine, the findings do support the experiences of many people: that foods rich in glutamates play a role in headaches.

In looking at this EAAT2 gene, another interesting fact emerges. Scientists at Ohio State University researching irritable bowel syndrome (IBS) found that, by doubling the amount of the EAAT2 protein in experimental mice, they could significantly reduce abdominal pain.[30] As a migraine attack is often associated with abdominal symptoms, and the presence of migraine in a patient is a marker for an increased risk of IBS, the finding is significant. (The same research group also made a link to the more serious problem of irritable bowel disorder.) EAAT2 has previously been associated with other illnesses, such as epilepsy, schizophrenia, and mood and anxiety disorders. So it seems that the more we learn, the more we need to learn!

If this gene has a message for us, it must be to look closely at the foods we eat, and especially at food additives, such as MSG. For some people, these ingredients may be no problem, but for those who suspect that their headaches have a link to food, this information may help them in choosing a diet from the later chapters.

Genes associated with familial common migraine (MA and MO)

Since at least 1998, genetic studies have suggested a link between the clinical presence of migraine and the X chromosome. In 2011, a Norfolk Island study that focused on this sex chromosome found a link to familial common migraine.[31] As women get two copies of the X chromosome, this finding may offer another explanation for the increased frequency, and often the increased severity, of migraine in women. Furthermore, the authors of the study make the same observation that many doctors have: the hormonal influences seem to work in either direction. Migraine may improve or deteriorate with the onset of puberty, menopause, or pregnancy, or with the use of oral contraceptives.

Genes associated with familial hemiplegic migraine (FHM)

Familial hemiplegic migraine is a particularly nasty form of migraine. It is relatively uncommon, but it was one of the earliest headaches to be clearly identified as genetically based because the case histories followed a Mendelian dominant pattern of inheritance. It will be discussed further in Chapter 10. For our purposes here, it is enough to say that the genes involved may explain why diets that more closely reflect the balance of sodium to potassium, and magnesium to calcium, in the natural world may help some headache sufferers.

Genes associated with cluster headaches

Cluster headaches are a distinctive form of headache. Relatively rare, they are far more common in males than females. They are regarded as the severest of all headaches, earning them the ominous title of 'suicide headaches'.

Sharing some similarities with migraine, cluster headaches are described as 'neurovascular primary headaches, involving the hypothalamic and trigeminovascular systems'. These are medical terms for the anatomical location, and the mechanism of the pain. The terms are described in more detail in Chapter 11. Inflammatory and immunological pathways are assumed to be part of the headache activation.

The ADH4 variant: a gene that helps to explain the link between alcohol and cluster headache

An association with alcohol consumption is a feature of cluster headaches, so some researchers set about looking at genetic differences in how people metabolise alcohol. Alcohol has to be detoxified through one of two pathways. Most of it goes via enzymes known as the alcohol dehydrogenases, or ADHs. Humans have seven ADH genes clustered on chromosome 4. Of these, the ADH4 gene helps us deal with vitamin A, steroids, and biogenic amines. It is a polymorphic gene, and one variant was found to be strongly associated with cluster headaches, especially if the person carried two copies of it.

Genes associated with tension headache, migraine, and jaw disorders

While I regard migraine as the most debilitating of all types of headache, others would put more emphasis on tension headaches because they are so common. The International Headache Society declares that it is the most common cause of primary headache, with a lifetime prevalence, in studies quoted by the society, of 30 to 78 per cent. Prevalence at any one point in time is much less than that. Previously known by names such as 'ordinary headache', 'stress headache', and 'psychogenic headache', the agreed terminology now is 'tension-type headache'. This headache is now thought to have a neurobiological basis, and, not surprisingly, some genetic associations have been identified. Some of these associations overlap with those for other kinds of headache. Tension-type headache is discussed more fully in Chapter 10.

CALCA gene

Various genes have been studied in relation to chronic tension headaches. One is the CALCA gene on chromosome 11. The CALCA gene codes for a protein called calcitonin gene-related peptide, or CGRP. This is a peptide made up of 37 amino acids. It causes dilation of cerebral blood vessels, which could account for the pounding or throbbing experienced with some headaches. It also seems to have a role in passing on pain messages.

This peptide has also been studied in the context of migraine, other headaches, and temporo-mandibular joint disorders — where it is found to be present in high levels. It is released from neurones in the trigeminal ganglion. From there it binds to CGRP receptors, causing blood vessels to dilate, and mast cells to degranulate (when certain white cells, called 'mast cells', become reactive, they release inflammatory chemicals, including histamine, in a process known as 'degranulation').[32] So if you have a particular vulnerable polymorphism of this gene, you may have an increased risk of all these types of headache.

But your problems may not stop there. Carriers of certain alleles have been shown to have almost double the risk of essential hypertension.[33]

SERT: a gene that might explain the link between headaches and mood disorders

Serotonin is a neurotransmitter. Its role in headache, headache-related disorders, and medications to treat them will be discussed throughout. SERT is the serotonin-transporter protein gene, found on chromosome 17. It has been studied in connection with migraine and chronic tension headaches.

The protein is the target of the SSRI antidepressant drugs. (See more on SSRIs in Chapters 9 and 13.) Some polymorphisms in the SERT gene affect the rate of serotonin uptake. They have been linked to conditions as varied as alcoholism, depression, obsessive–compulsive disorder, hypertension, social phobia, and even cot death. Fascinating recent research asserts that this gene has two key variants, called the short form and the long form.[34] As we all get one variant from each parent, we might have a short/short, a long/long, or a short/long combination. People with a long/long genotype seem to be protected from depression. Moreover, of the apes, only humans and rhesus monkeys have any short versions at all. On the upside, the short versions seem to go with adaptability, emotional responsiveness, and good communication and social skills.

The link between SERT and headache has been studied in the context of short and long versions of the gene, but it will be interesting to see if headache turns out to be *genetically* linked to mood.[35]

Other genes

You mean there's more, doctor? Many other genes impact on your overall risk of headache. Some are discussed in Chapter 10.

HOW DOES GENETIC INFORMATION HELP ME TO MANAGE MY HEADACHES?

Now that we have looked at some of the known genetic factors linked to headache, let us return to our hypothetical consultation of the future in which you and I looked at your genome together. I have gone through your profile and found that you have several weak spots for headaches.

What do you do now? Throw in the towel and decide to leave your faulty body to science? Get depressed and ask me for some Prozac? Or do we set out to minimise harm so that, jointly, we can ensure that your risk of future headaches is reduced? If you have inherited an unfortunate gene, that's bad luck. If you have two or three, it may be very bad luck. But if you have inherited a whole raft of 'bad' genes, maybe we have our paradigm wrong. A lot of these seemingly unfortunate genes may be the very genes that gave our species its robustness. In the animal world it's called 'hybrid vigour'.

You can see from what you have already read about these genes that dietary inputs may increase or reduce their impact. Is there enough folic acid and vitamin B12 in your diet to support your more-vulnerable genes? Are you low in vitamin D? Could a high-salt diet be contributing to your migraine? Would finding a drug for the migraine *pain* allow you to continue eating a dangerously high salt load, perhaps leading to heart attack and stroke?

And what about increased sensory stimuli? Could the acute sense of smell, which once might have allowed you to detect noxious gases from leaking volcanic vents, now be activated by the perfume department in the local department store, or the 'fragrance' in the powder room of the upmarket hotel, or the 'air freshener' in the doctor's surgery?

To make the point more forcefully: perhaps it's not *we* that are sick — it's our diet and our environment; our whole way of life.

A closer look at some of these genes

You will see some, though not all, of the genes in Diagram 1 on page 50 are represented as black panels with white lettering. You can see where the folic acid in our diet is heading, and how it is linked to the production of serotonin and dopamine. A roadblock in the folic-acid cycle may represent a roadblock in the adjacent cycles. The MTHFR polymorphism we have discussed represents one such roadblock. To have a double dose of this gene variant makes for an even bigger one. But we saw that B6, B12, and folic acid all support this gene, and Lyn Griffiths' work gives us a simple non-drug treatment we can try.

If we have a copy of the 'wrong' variant of the ACE gene, we might do well to look at how much salt we eat, not only for our headaches but also to avoid a rise in blood pressure, increased cortisol production, and stress. At the bottom of this diagram we see where glutamate makes its appearance. Will it go to calming GABA on the right, or to increased neuronal agitation (and headache) on the left?

Look at where the letters 'VDR' are located. This refers to the type of vitamin D receptors you inherit. If they are a less efficient version, you might need more than average amounts of vitamin D to make dopamine (the feel-good hormone), and so on.

Learning from genetics

I had been ordering MTHFR gene tests on migraine patients for a couple of years without ever thinking that I might test my own. After all, I had already put in place many of the strategies that are outlined in Chapter 8, and they had worked; my headaches were rare by now, and pretty mild. I had endured and survived *hyperemesis gravidarum* in my pregnancies. Despite a lean build, I was hypertensive, but that was probably due to work stress. I knew I should slow down because I still ran the risk of post-menopausal stroke, but such general indications were easy to ignore.

Then a couple of things happened. I got a viral inner-ear infection (labyrinthitis), had a mini-stroke, and my blood pressure became difficult to control.

So I decided to do this one gene test, knowing that the cost was not huge. When the results came back, I stared in disbelief. I was homozygous for (had two copies of) one of the most significant migraine genes.

And there was more. Further gene studies showed that I had two copies of the undesirable MTRR variant, and two copies of an undesirable form of a gene called MAO A. We have not discussed MAO A here, but it is another gene on the X chromosome. It affects our ability to control neurotransmitters such as serotonin, and it has been linked to migraine. (Drugs relating to serotonin control in migraine are discussed in Chapter 9.)

But if I were designer-made to experience migraine, I was also homozygous for the deleterious ACE D polymorphism, and homozygous for the unfortunate vitamin D receptor polymorphisms.

Nowadays, if I saw anyone with genes like these, I would recommend adequate vitamin D levels, vitamin B12, (natural) folic acid, and vitamin B6. I always recommend magnesium. I see no harm in suggesting these nutrients anyway. I wish I had known all this in the years during which I was plagued by headaches.

CHAPTER 3
The Bullets: foods that can produce headache

'However beautiful the strategy, you should occasionally look at the results ... Man will occasionally stumble over the truth, but most of the time he will pick himself up and continue on.'
WINSTON CHURCHILL

I met Grainne because she and her partner ran an excellent secondhand bookshop that I, and many bibliophiles, loved to frequent. It seemed as if no quality title, however obscure, could escape a place on their shelves, or could evade being tracked down by them.

One day while I was in the shop, I learned that Grainne had gone home with a migraine, and that this was not uncommon. Learning of my interest in this area, she later consulted me, and agreed that although running the shop was very rewarding, the hours were long. Often her meals consisted of homemade soup. We discussed the fact that she had given up smoking, both out of concern for her health and because she had felt that smoking was a migraine trigger.

Having given up, her general health had improved, but there had been little impact on the headaches.

I recommended that Grainne undertake an elimination diet. As a vegetarian, she had based many of her soups on tomato extract. After she eliminated this, the headaches improved, but they did not disappear.

The second time around, my questioning became more focused — and I was taken aback to learn that she was continually snacking on liquorice allsorts. Always a favourite, they had become almost a substitute addiction when she gave up smoking. The range of food colourings in these candies is impressive; they include almost all the suspect colours we will discuss shortly. So the tomatoes had gone, the liquorice allsorts went … and then, so did the headaches.

Many trials have examined the role of diet in headache, and many patients tell us they suspect a food connection. Some headache patients also suffer bowel problems such as irritable bowel, pointing to involvement of the digestive system. The name 'hot-dog headache' recognises a specific type of food-related headache, and it is widely known that red wine and chocolate can contribute to migraine. But apart from such examples, food reactions are not given a lot of consideration in the headache story. Many different attempts have been made to tackle headaches with diet. Some have been highly successful; others have failed, for reasons that may become apparent as we proceed.

IS IT SOMETHING I EAT?

It is obvious from Grainne's story that I think the answer is yes. Of course there are many provisos, such as 'depending on which genes you carry' and 'depending on what else is going on in your life'. What I'm saying is that the gun poses little threat if it has no bullets in it. And even if it is fully loaded, unless the trigger is pulled, it should remain safe. I see the 'bullets' as being mostly the common, everyday foods we eat. I will first look at some common foods and explain how the immune system works. Then I go on to look at the chemicals, both natural and synthetic, in food.

Some interesting studies involving common foods

We begin with the story of an impressive dietary trial. To my way of thinking, it should have transformed the management of migraine, but many arguments have been put forward to dispute this kind of work. Writings of neurologists such as Oliver Sacks and James Lance seem to minimise the effects of diet, but patients often suspect a dietary link. So what is the thinking here?

In the early 1980s, some neurologists at the Great Ormond Street Hospital in London undertook a seminal trial on the management of migraine in children.[36] One of these doctors felt that common foods were the basis of many of the migraines they were seeing. Elimination of such foods, he reasoned, would bring relief. The other four doctors were sceptical, but agreed to take part in the trial. The importance of this is that the trial was set up by a team of people who — with one notable exception — expected it to *fail*. In any trial, we know that the investigator's expectation is a significant predictor of outcome. This is not a comment on the integrity of the researchers — just a known fact of clinical trials. The results tend to bias towards the expectations of the researchers.

The Great Ormond Street trial enrolled 88 children aged from three to 16 who fitted the trial criteria — recurrent headaches accompanied by two of: nausea, abdominal pain, photophobia (sensitivity to light), visual disturbance, or weakness. The children were put on an elimination diet for four weeks. They were allowed one meat (usually lamb or chicken), one carbohydrate (rice or potato), one fruit (banana or apple), one vegetable (from the cabbage family), and some vitamins. Once two headache-free weeks had elapsed, normal foods were reintroduced, one at a time.

After the provoker foods had been identified, the children went back on the restricted diet, but were divided into two groups. One group had hidden traces of their provoking food included in their meals; the others did not. Foods were blended to taste the same, and put in cans. The study took several months.

The doctors did not know which group was which. Indeed, the whole trial conformed to the double-blind model, as the participants and their parents did not know whether the test food was 'spiked' or not. Only five of the mothers thought they could tell the difference between the 'trial' and the 'safe' foods, and only two of them were correct.

The results were startling. Those in the experimental arm of the study relapsed when traces of the culprit foods were reintroduced, whereas those still on safe foods did not. Then the two groups were swapped so that the opposite situation prevailed. Of the children who completed the diet, 93 per cent made either a complete or almost-complete recovery when eating foods safe for them. It has to be stressed that these children did not remain on the highly restrictive diet long term; their ongoing diet only removed the foods to which they had shown a reaction.

The findings

In this study, milk was by far the most common food provoking headaches. The number of children reacting to each food was: cow's milk, 27; egg, 24; chocolate, 22; orange, 21; wheat, 21; benzoic acid (E210–19), 14; cheese, 13; tomato, 13; tartrazine (E102), 12; rye, 12; fish, 9; pork, 9; beef, 8; maize, 8; soya, 7; tea, 7; oats, 6; goat's milk, 6; coffee, 6; peanuts, 5; bacon, 4; potato, 4; yeast, 4.

Clearly, many children reacted to more than one food. Indeed, the average number of reactive foods for any child was three.

Another interesting thing about this study is that before it had begun, neither the parents nor the children, though they may have suspected a food connection, had been able to predict which foods might be their culprit foods. It would have been reasonable to assume that people were suspicious of culprit foods, but as the authors of the study commented, it could take between one hour and seven days for the adverse reaction to occur, making identification tricky.

Is there a blood test for this?

It would be convenient for everyone if there were a simple blood test to determine adverse food reactions. There are several tests we can do, but the situation is not simple.

Let us start with the standard approach to 'allergy'. When we have an allergic reaction to something, such as a bee sting, a food, or a pollen, our body produces an immune globulin, a type of protein, called IgE. The 'Ig' stands for 'immune globulin'. The type of reaction in this case is referred to as 'E'. An IgE test is the routine blood or skin-prick test your doctor will do for 'true' allergy. More on this presently.

In about 1980, and just before the Great Ormond Street trial, Doctor Jean Monro at the National Hospital for Nervous Diseases in London was also investigating food sensitivities and headaches. She too used elimination diets, with some success.[37] She and her team wondered about blood tests. They found that although IgE testing was useful, the results were not very predictive. In the Great Ormond Street study, the IgE results similarly indicated that only three children would have recovered if IgE testing on its own had been relied on.

For migraine, it seemed, we needed a better test. The elimination diet gave useful answers, but required considerable effort.

In the absence of a simple, reliable test, it was hard to convince the medical fraternity of a link between food and headache. With doctors refuting the connection, and patients themselves unable to predict problematic foods, it is not hard to see why the idea did not catch on. Even now, although some people suspect a food link to their headaches, many find it confusing. Some will say, 'But it can't be orange juice, doctor; I have orange juice every morning but I only get the headaches twice a month.' Or, 'It can't be milk; I only have milk at breakfast but I always get my headaches at night.' On first contact with the concept, I too used all of these arguments.

Why isn't it obvious?
The difficulty in identifying culprit foods may arise from several factors:

- more than one food may be involved
- the response may be delayed
- the response may be dose-related
- the response may be intermittent, based on what else is happening in the person's life, such as the timing of the female menstrual cycle.

This is not the way most of us intuitively think. We tend to think that if something makes us ill, we will know straight away, and that is understandable. However, it is regrettable for medical professionals to limit their thinking in this way.

SOME IMMUNOLOGY

To understand what is happening here, it is important to come to grips with some aspects of the immune system. This is not complex science, so please do not be put off.

Broadly speaking, the immune system developed to fight germs. Over time, it has come to fight not only germs but also pollens, foods, food additives, pollutants, and injected materials, such as stings, venoms, and vaccines.

It is convenient to compare our immune system to a nation's defence forces. When the immune system is alerted to potential danger, it has several options. For one, it can react through its primitive pathways to 'seek and destroy'. White cells such as phagocytes can simply swallow the enemy. Primitive? Yes. Effective? Very. This aspect of the immune system is sometimes referred to as the 'innate' immune system.

Apart from swallowing the enemy, the primitive immune system also has chemical warfare at its disposal. Certain cells — epithelial cells in the gut or mast cells in the blood — may 'poison' the enemy with nitric oxide, serotonin, histamine, or other chemicals. If this seems an odd reaction to food, remember that the prime job of a responsive immune system was to fight germs, but now it has broadened its scope. So a defence mechanism that might have killed a germ is now warning us off a food by giving us prickly skin or a headache. And of course, the message may be obscured if there is a long delay.

So the innate immune system can destroy or poison substances that threaten it. Over time, as higher animals evolved, they developed more sophisticated immune responses. Specific immune cells — B lymphocytes, to be precise — learned to make targeted immune globulins. We have already looked at immune globulin type E, IgE. This targeted aspect of the immune system is referred to as the 'adaptive' immune system.

These immune globulins fall into one of five classes, known as IgE, IgG, IgA, IgM, and IgD. On contact with the 'enemy', the B lymphocytes produce an immune complex using 'data', or immune memory gained from previous encounters. The defining characteristics of an intact adaptive immune system are just that: immune *specificity* and *memory*.

For our purposes here, we need to look at only three immune globulins: IgE, IgG, and IgA.

IgE reactions

Reactions produced by IgE are immediate, and are often in response to foods, stings, and inhalants like pollens. This might seem removed from the original brief of fighting germs, but the immediate responses of IgE reactions can include sneezing, vomiting, or diarrhoea — efficient ways of getting rid of something that is toxic to us. The immediacy of the response leaves little doubt about the connection between cause and effect. Most IgE reactions are mild, but there is one exception to this: anaphylaxis.

Anaphylaxis is life-threatening. Symptoms include an itchy rash, swelling in the throat, and low blood pressure. Sufferers have to carry adrenalin (an EpiPen) with them at all times, because the effects can kill. IgE reactions ensure attention from the medical profession because they can be so dangerous. The most common foods involved are peanuts, sesame, prawns, and crustaceans, but any food may trigger such a reaction. The risk from bee and wasp stings is also well known. Over time, doctors have come to use the term 'allergic' when referring to IgE reactions, whether they result in anaphylaxis or not.

IgG reactions

In contrast to IgE, IgG is about long-term memory. As part of its brief to fight germs, the IgG arm of the immune system gives us a long-term memory for previous infection. This is why we can fight germs that we have met before, and it is the reason that we become 'immune' to certain infections after we have had them once.

But here too the immune system has widened its scope beyond germs, and now embraces foods. Such reactions may have an adverse effect on us. And because the IgG reactions are *delayed*, an IgG food reaction may not be immediately apparent. If we go back to our migraineurs, it would be reasonable to consider that a food eaten today could evoke an IgG-based headache three days later. Because IgG reactions do not kill, they currently receive much less attention from doctors. Indeed, many doctors, taking IgE as the only cause of 'true' allergy, scoff at the idea that IgG reactions may be any sort of a problem at all. However, that view is changing.

Another link to irritable bowel syndrome
In Chapter 2, we looked at a gene possibly connecting migraine with irritable bowel syndrome. In the United Kingdom, tests for IgG food reactions have shown benefit in deciding which foods might be eliminated in the management of IBS.[38] Shortly we shall read of a study where IgG testing enabled management of colitis (inflammation of the lower bowel), a condition closely linked to IBS. This bowel condition is important in its own right, but we should note that it often occurs in headache sufferers. Many remark that change in bowel habit is part of the prodroma (early symptoms) of a headache. 'My bowels turn to water, and that's how I know a headache is coming on' is a lament that I have sometimes heard.

Some recent research has contributed to the case for the involvement of IgG food reactions in migraine. In 2005, nearly 40 years after the original Great Ormond Street and Monro studies, a small pilot study in the United Kingdom recruited 61 'high-impact' migraine patients.[39] Blood tests for IgG food antibodies were taken, and appropriate diets advised. Forty-six patients completed one month on the diet, and 39 completed two months. After one month of avoiding their IgG reactants, 27.5 per cent reported considerable benefit, and 30 per cent reported little or no benefit. At two months, 38.2 per cent reported considerable benefit, and 32.4 per cent reported little or none. The remainder reported benefits in between these two extremes.

The foods reacted to, in order of frequency, were: cow's milk, yeast, egg white, egg yolk, wheat, gliadin, corn, cashew, mollusc mix, brazil nuts, cranberry, and garlic. The overlap with the findings of the Great Ormond Street study is significant. The average number of foods reacted to was 4.7, with a range from 1 to 17.

Another study was carried out in Mexico, with the laboratory analyses done in a Fort Lauderdale laboratory in the United States.[40] After skin-prick tests for IgE allergy, and blood tests for IgG reactions, the 56 subjects — all migraine sufferers — were placed on a six-month elimination diet specific to their individual results. A control group (non-migraineurs) had similar blood tests carried out. Positive IgG food reactions were found in *all* of the migraineurs, and 26 per cent of the control group. The number of foods to which the migraineurs reacted on the IgG tests ranged from six to 30, and in the control group, from none to four. The foods most likely to cause a reaction were: banana, beans, cheese, cow's milk, eggs, mushroom, sugar, wheat, and yeast. Close behind these were tomatoes, pork, chilli, oranges, lemon, corn, peanuts, and prawns. Once again, the overlap with foods in the studies already discussed is striking.

In only three cases was the IgE reactivity similar to the IgG results. Reactivity in each case seemed far greater in terms of IgG than IgE ratings.

By sticking to the diet over the six-month period, 43 subjects experienced no migraine at all, four reported a decrease in intensity and frequency, and nine reported no change. These results were deemed to be statistically significant to a high probability level.

An interesting finding from the study was that six of the subjects also had a diagnosis of colitis. After one month on the special diet, both conditions had improved.

Does this mean I'm allergic to those foods?

As we have seen, the term 'allergy' generally applies to IgE reactions. Because these food reactions are based on IgG responses, they are not allergies. In the past, we called them 'food intolerances', but the current trend is to call them 'non-allergic food hypersensitivities'. These semantic niceties seem to keep doctors happy. The patients just want to know whether it is worth avoiding certain foods.

Should I get these tests done?

If you suspect that some foods are implicated in your headaches, it may be useful to get a blood test for IgG reactions. The test will cost several hundred dollars; it does not usually attract any rebate within the healthcare system, but some private funds support such testing. I do not know of any publicly funded clinics in Australia that have even done trials testing IgG food reactions. Sadly, the opinion still seems to be that the tests contribute little to the understanding of migraine or other headaches. Hopefully, the weight of evidence will eventually change this. After all, not even the much-lauded triptan medications produce results as good as those seen in the trials that we have just been looking at.

Admittedly, the authors of one of the above studies comment that 'the mechanisms of IgG food mediated allergy have not been fully elucidated and remain speculative'. They speculate that mast cells may be activating T helper and B lymphocytes to put out more IgG antibodies and cytokines, which then lead to an inflammatory response.[41]

The details of reliable laboratories providing IgG testing are in Appendix 2. If the cost of the tests is beyond your means, an elimination diet is even more reliable, and it's free. It's just more tedious to do!

IgA reactions

The third immune globulin relevant to our discussion is IgA. IgA antibodies can be found circulating in the bloodstream, and also in the secretions from the mucosa, where it is known as secretory IgA, or sIgA. Secretory IgA antibodies can be found in colostrum, breast milk, tears, saliva, digestive juices, and fluid in the genito-urinary tract. For our purposes, IgA antibodies are most relevant in the detection of gluten intolerance and coeliac disease. Indeed, IgA reactions constitute the fundamental diagnostic test for this disease.

Many people who have a problem with gluten also suffer headaches. Some lose their migraines once they become gluten-free. It is probable that if we could do IgA testing for the same range of foods as we can with IgG food reactions, we would identify another group of 'non-allergic food sensitivities' borne by the headache patient.

Selective IgA deficiency can exist either as an inherited or an acquired deficiency. In this case, recurrent infection is a common outcome, including chronic sinusitis and urinary tract infections. These people also seem to exhibit more adverse reactions to foods.

Food families

Tests for IgE or IgG usually examine about 100 or so foods. However, this does not cover the whole range of foods that go into our mouths, and sometimes it is helpful to remove other foods from the same family. The food-family chart in Appendix 1 is useful here. For me, mangoes, cashew nuts, and pistachios were always problematic. All of these plants come from the same botanical family (*Anacardiaceae*). It is common to find people reacting to a whole range of foods from one food family.

Milk and migraine

We have just seen that milk is one of the most reactive foods for migraine sufferers; it is frequently associated with irritable bowel syndrome as well. Let us look at another patient.

We met Catherine in Chapter 1: she was the professional musician whose career had been threatened by recurrent migraine. She had been seen by more than one specialist, but did not feel that her headaches were under control. So we began the all-purpose elimination diet, and by the second or third headache-free menstrual cycle, she was convinced.

Catherine liked milky coffee (so many migraineurs seem to!), and indeed, when under duress, had seemed to get by on lattes and cappucinos. But she was determined to stick to the diet. Some time after giving up her fix, she volunteered that on one occasion she had broken out and had a latte, which 'came up as fast as it went down'. It seemed that milk was the major 'bullet' for Catherine, and, with a few other minor dietary adjustments, she seemed to be doing very well. In my mind, we had removed the bullets, so the gun gave Catherine no trouble. Unfortunately, as we shall see in Chapter 6, it isn't always that simple.

FOOD CHEMICALS AND ADDITIVES

'There's no such a thing as junk food.' This statement comes from a food scientist. Her position was simple: there's food and there's junk.

So now we leave immunology and turn to what goes into our mouths. The diet in the Great Ormond Street study removed all food additives, and there were good reasons for this. Although some children showed evidence of an IgE reaction to some of the additives, many of the reactions were not caused by 'allergy' or immune globulin reactions of any kind.

Adverse food reactions do not have to be a reaction to a complex food protein, like 'cow's milk' or 'peanuts'. Sometimes the body may be reacting to one of the simple molecules found in nature, such as a phenol, a salicylate, or an amine. These molecules are part of the food, and it may be them, rather than the whole food, that causes the adverse reaction. So when we react to the peanut or the milk, we still need to consider which part of the food is responsible.

Such thinking has led over time to various hypotheses, the best known of which is the 'amine hypothesis'. Substances such as phenols, salicylates, and amines exist in the plant world as part of the plant's defence mechanism. These natural chemicals may act as an insecticide, a fungicide, or a pesticide, or they may act as an antioxidant to protect the plant from the ultraviolet radiation of the sun. In short, they may be part of the plant's own 'immune system'.

We have just seen that humans (along with other vertebrates) have a couple of levels of immune defence: the innate and the adaptive immune systems. The plant has to make do with its innate immune system alone. It does this through the production of simple chemicals, such as salicylic acid, to ward off microbial attack. Indeed, one of the genes for disease resistance in plants is known as 'salicylic acid–binding protein 2'.[42] Further understanding of plant defence came from the Klessig research group,[43] with the discovery of a plant gene for nitric oxide synthase, the enzyme that rapidly produces nitric oxide after infection. This is one of the earliest responses by the plant to pathogen attack. As we shall soon see, it plays a significant role in our story too.

Messenger molecules

You may have recognised some familiar names here. Phenols, salicylates, and amines (discussed in some detail in Chapter

12) are some of the very molecules involved in the headache pathways in humans.

As part of our 'immune defence' against foreign invaders, people, like plants, produce some simple chemicals that act as messenger molecules. And because we are all genetically different, each of us has different targets and different degrees of response to things seen by our bodies as 'foreign'. Headache is just one of those responses. Not only are we producing some of the molecules ourselves, but we are also ingesting them in our food. Our diet, our digestion, our genetic makeup — all of these things will determine whether we respond with a headache, an asthma attack, or seemingly no response at all, whenever 'self' recognises 'non-self'. Of course, we respond to our environment every second of every day — it's just that most of our responses go unnoticed because most of them cause us no problem.

When one part of the body wants to communicate with another, the easiest way is via a messenger molecule. This messenger gets into the bloodstream and travels around until it gets to the target organ, where it docks onto a receptor site and delivers its message. Or it can use another highway. If neurons in your brain want to talk to your big toe, they do not use the bloodstream; instead, they use nerves to send electrical messages down until they reach your toe. Involved in the initiation and delivery of this process are some other messenger molecules, the neurotransmitters. You will probably be familiar with some names for these messenger molecules, such as 'hormones' and 'neurotransmitters'; other names are 'cytokines' (small proteins) and 'inflammatory chemicals'.

Food as drugs

If we wonder why certain foods can have such profound effects on us, it may help to think of them as drugs. Mother Nature is economical. Rather than dreaming up many new molecules to do various jobs, she presses into service the molecules she has already used for building the rest of the biological world. At the simplest level, this means that food that tastes nice is food that sends a pleasurable message to our brain. Hopefully this ensures that we keep eating nutritious foods, and thus our species will survive.

In the botanical world, a plant that has tasty fruits and flowers attracts birds and bees, which disseminate seeds and pollen, so that the species will survive. But the tree does not want its fruit to be eaten up before the seed is mature, so it incorporates repellant features while the fruit is green. In the case of green fruit, high salicylate levels help make the fruit unattractive and, as we have seen above, salicylic acid also repels disease. As the fruit matures, it changes colour and develops sugars, because now Mother Nature wants the fruit to be eaten.

Nature's blueprints

If we stay with the 'food as drug' idea, what is it about certain foods that have a pharmacological or drug-like effect on us? Many modern drugs imitate hormones, neurotransmitters, or cytokines; other drugs are designed to block the action of one of these natural substances. When manufacturers create a drug, they want it to achieve what our body is trying to achieve and cannot, or what our diet should achieve and does not; or they want it to block what our body is doing when it should not (often because of factors such as poor diet). In doing so, drug manufacturers rely on nature's blueprints.

Because we share a lot of our biochemistry with plants, molecules such as nitric oxide operate in plants and in ourselves. Plants make nitric oxide, and so do we. Salicylates are not only part of a plant defence mechanism; they also have an effect on our nervous system. The fact that in 2011 some experts were still trying to resolve the question of whether mushrooms are plants or animals surely makes the point that we have more than a little in common with the plant world.

So in summary, many molecules that nature is using for a pharmacological purpose in plants have a pharmacological effect on us. And often that effect is similar to that of a hormone, a neurotransmitter, or a cytokine. We accept the negative consequences of being 'drugged' like this in return for the many benefits food confers upon us. (Like staying alive, for example!)

Foods most commonly seen as drug-like are gluten and milk. This is because of their breakdown products, gluteomorphin from gluten and caseomorphin from milk. The relationship to morphine, the product of another natural substance, is unmistakable linguistically and chemically. They are often referred to as 'opioid' foods. And indeed, people find them very addictive. Most of the Western diet is based on them, after all. When scientists learn from nature to make drugs and develop chemicals for agricultural purposes or food preservation, the outcome for us is not always benign. Many pesticides and fungicides affect our biochemistry. They work because they *can* mess with the biology of insects and plants. In humans, they might become known as a 'gender bender' or an 'endocrine disruptor', and they can affect our biology or reproductive capacity in a negative way. Preservatives act by killing microbes, also known as 'germs'. But what happens to the good microbes that inhabit our intestines and make up a significant part of our immune system? And what happens to those people who cannot easily detoxify these chemicals? We have all inherited enzymes suitable to life in the rainforest, ill equipped to cope with a 21st-century chemical load.

These many chemicals are employed as preservatives, colourants, 'flavour enhancers', pesticides, fungicides, and the like. The unfortunate side effects for health are often accepted by 'experts' as 'tolerable' levels of collateral damage.

Chapters 12 and 13 look at some of these molecules in depth. Here I will just make the observation that they divide into two groups, nature's and synthetic molecules. The division, however, is somewhat arbitrary.

Nature's molecules
Chemicals in this list include many that will be familiar to most of us. The words 'histamine', 'serotonin', and 'dopamine' have become part of everyday language. Others, such as 'caffeine', always were. All of these compounds can be classified as biologically active amines. Yet others, such as 'salicylates', are becoming part of common parlance. Salicylates are a different group of chemicals to amines, but are more of 'nature's blueprints'.

Synthetic molecules

Many ingredients are added to commercially prepared food. A quick check of the ingredient list on the packaging of an item as simple as bread or biscuits makes this clear. Food scientists, over the years, have drawn on nature's blueprints in creating these additives. The purpose may be for food colouration or preservation. They may perform some action such as leavening bread, or be an 'anti-caking' agent. The unintended effects on humans include behavioural changes, headaches, or related conditions, such as abdominal pain. I believe that it is not always easy to separate these as distinct pathologies.

In summary: problem foods

A systematic approach to choosing an elimination diet is discussed in Chapter 6. But for now, here are some standout culprits:

- caffeine
- citrus
- chocolate
- corn
- egg
- dairy products
- food additives and colours
- mushrooms
- peanuts and other nuts
- soy
- sugar
- tomato
- wheat, rye, and other gluten cereals
- yeast (and the yeast extract some love on their toast).

For many years, the Feingold Diet, which purported to help children suffering from attention-deficit disorders, was dismissed as invalid. When *The Lancet* published a UK study, led by Professor Jim Stevenson, that showed an adverse effect of food colours on children, many people felt that Feingold had finally been vindicated.[44] The details of this study appear in Chapter 12.

So as we conclude this survey of some of the main bullets, the argument is simple: unload the gun where possible, and a headache will be less likely to occur.

CHAPTER 4
The Triggers: what can set off the headache gun

'Scientific apparatus offer a window to knowledge, but as they grow more elaborate, scientists spend ever more time washing the windows.'
Isaac Asimov

I saw Iris again a few months after her initial contact. She does not smoke and does not drink. Genetic tests for a 'migraine gene' (MTHFR; see Chapter 2) had been positive, and she had been 'putting locks' on her triggers (see Chapter 8) by taking magnesium and B-group vitamins for several months.

When she first came to me, she said she hoped that menopause would be the end of her headaches, but it had brought no relief. Now she was desperate, and was travelling a long way to see me. She said that she would do anything to prevent the constant cycle of headaches, and all the medication she needs to take for them. She had tried an elimination diet, which takes a lot of determination. I thought we had a good strategy. So why wasn't she getting better?

Her headaches were waking her around three or four in the morning. She woke very nauseous and already wanting to vomit. It seemed that she had been faithful to the diet, but had been unable to give up her daily six or more cups of strong tea. Because the headaches were persisting, she had continued to use Naramig (a triptan, see Chapter 9) three or four times a week. It was not hard to figure out what was going on here: medication overuse was compounding the headaches.

In situations like this, an elimination diet was really a bit premature, like trying to fix a smoker's cough while the person is still smoking. Iris had two serious addictions: the caffeine in the tea, and Naramig. By 3 a.m., her body was ready for its 'fix' and was in withdrawal.

We began a careful weaning process of both. This had to be done slowly, and Iris had to endure several very unpleasant headaches along the way. There was some progress: after a while her headaches were less debilitating, but they were not cured. She decided to take extra steps, doing some of the peripheral things that we will discuss shortly. She had a neck massage, which she felt was a breakthrough. Modern thinking on headache entirely supports this.[45]

So Iris was getting a handle on several things. She was reducing the addictive drugs; reducing the dietary 'bullets'; taking the nutritional supports; and obtaining relief of muscle tension, a probable trigger.

Now, some time later, Iris rarely uses headache pills anymore. She has resumed drinking tea, but intersperses caffeinated varieties with herbal teas and water. It is hard to separate cause from effect, but her feeling that she has some control over her headaches must also have contributed to the lessening of their occurrence.

COMMON CAUSES OF HEADACHE

In the previous chapter, I discussed the foods that might load the 'bullets' into the genetic headache 'gun'. That approach has all the weaknesses of an argument by analogy, but let us stick with it and turn our attention to triggers.

Many patients that I see have some idea about what sets their headaches off, but an equal number do not. Even if they eat the same foods every day, some days are headache-free, and on other days, bed is the only place to be. This is not surprising because the triggers can be subtle. Let's look at some of them.

Stress

I begin with stress because that's where headache sufferers usually begin their story. Invariably they tell me that the headaches are worse during times of stress. Some people take extreme steps, such as changing jobs, or even taking early retirement. Others try simpler solutions, such as practising yoga and meditation.

All such options are worth consideration, but for some people the luxury of changing their job is just not possible. For example, as the wife of a senior politician, Cindy McCain's destiny was essentially mapped out; she was a public figure whether she liked it or not. Mothers with young families similarly lack choices. If money is tight, or if they are single parents, even a yoga course is a luxury they cannot afford. Better solutions must be found.

Relaxation

Ironically, just as stress and muscle tension can trigger a headache, so too can relaxation. See 'Friday nights' on page 104.

Muscle tension

Most headache sufferers at some point mention neck pain and stiffness, or teeth clenching and grinding. This subject was introduced in Chapter 1, and we discuss it further in the next chapter.

Chapter 11 looks at muscle tension in the context of tension-type headaches, and dental contributions to headache. The question of cause and effect is relevant here. Many of my patients have benefited from interventions as simple as muscle-relaxation exercises or a dental brace. Iris certainly identified the neck massage as a breakthrough.

New research has focused on the occipital nerve, because it feeds directly into the brain circuits associated with migraine. A connection is likely, given the number of people who comment on neck stiffness and pain as the warning sign for their headaches, or who are helped by neck massage.

Travel sickness

The potential for motion sickness is almost universal (except where the inner ear has been destroyed by disease or there is significant cerebellar disease). The literature linking migraine with travel sickness is extensive. Motion sickness is five times more common in migraineurs, and about 50 per cent of migraine sufferers identify it as a problem. In children, carsickness can be one of the first presentations of a migraine tendency.[46] Many migraine sufferers learn early that reading in a car is just not on.

Research conducted in 2005 by doctors Peter Drummond and Anna Granston concluded that head pain and motion sickness both activate the migraine mechanism independently, so that the inputs might intensify each other.[47] This is why the antihistamines used for migraine are also useful to prevent carsickness.

Lighting

Some migraineurs find that visual cues can trigger their headaches. Culprits include stripes, strobe lighting, and flickering fluorescent lights. Strobe lighting is used in nightclubs, but train drivers have reported a similar problem is caused as they pass through a rapid succession of tunnels and daylight.[48]

People often identify Picasso as a migraine sufferer because of the nature of the distortion in his paintings. Although he apparently never complained of headaches, individuals such as Michel Ferrari, a Dutch neurologist, claim that sketches by migraineurs, when asked to draw what they see during an attack, are 'extremely similar' to Picasso's work.[49] It is even possible that he belonged to a group whom we would today classify as 'aura-predominant migraine sufferers'. I have seen several such patients. The pain is minimal to absent, but visual distortion, sometimes accompanied by vertigo, can dominate their lives.

Picasso aside, the visual triggers raise questions of cause and effect. Does the headache cause the distortion, or do certain patterns trigger headaches? I suspect that it works both ways. Many patients find certain artworks or geometric patterns difficult to look at, inducing vertigo at the very least.

Headache sufferers readily identify flickering fluorescent lights as triggers. Energy-saving compact fluorescent lights can have this effect, even when the flicker is below a detectable threshold. Fluorescent lights have been increasingly associated with migraine and epilepsy.[50] The phasing-out of incandescent lights poses a problem for Australian migraine sufferers. Authorities in the United Kingdom have considered reintroducing incandescent lights on these health grounds.[51] LED lights are claimed to be superior to fluorescent lights because of the absence of flicker. However, they still emit significant electromagnetic radiation (EMR, discussed shortly), and have been associated with the triggering of headache in some people.

Compact fluorescent lights are frequently a bright blue-white colour. LEDs also emit light with a strong blue peak. This is a very narrow part of the electromagnetic spectrum, which is why they save energy, but they can impact upon melatonin levels.[52]

Sleep disturbance and melatonin levels

We know that lack of sleep predisposes people to headaches of all types. Melatonin, produced by the pineal gland, is the hormone that induces sleep. Melatonin is a small hormone with many effects; for example, it is a powerful antioxidant.

Both night work and sleeping during daylight hours

reduce the opportunity for the pineal gland to make melatonin. Low levels of melatonin may explain the finding that women who work regular night shifts have a 50 per cent increased risk of breast cancer.[53] Melatonin has been used to regulate the effects of circadian disruption in the migraine cascade.[54] It has also been advocated for chronic tension headache, cluster headache, and other types of headache.[55]

Melatonin production is switched off by bright light and light from the blue end of the colour spectrum. If your house is brightly lit with blue-white light until you go to bed, your melatonin production will fall. At least one study has shown that 'altered melatonin levels have been found in cluster headache, migraine with and without aura, menstrual migraine, and chronic migraine'.[56]

Soft, yellow-toned lighting in the evening, and meditation, can raise melatonin levels.

Perfume and other chemicals

On many occasions I have seen patients who have come to me because they know I am interested in headache. As they enter my room, I can smell the perfume and need to open a window to let the odour escape. I cannot believe that they have not made the connection between perfume and headache, but if you apply it every day, and the fumes are saturating your clothing, then it is akin to foods eaten daily. Why would you link them to headache?

From my perspective, perfume is only one of the many examples of a toxic petrochemical smog that surrounds us all, and I have to refrain from saying as much on first encounter. Such triggers are so important that I have devoted the whole of Chapter 7 to them. Other chemicals discussed in Chapter 7 include persistent organic pollutants (POPs), polycyclic aromatic hydrocarbons (PAHs), and cigarette smoke.

Certain foods

Foods notorious for causing headache include chocolate, red wine, citrus, and cheese. While I have said that these foods can act as bullets, the rapid reactions from some of them indicate that they are acting more like triggers. Food additives and colours can also have the rapid onset typical of a trigger, and the migraine literature frequently refers to them as such. Chapter 6 deals with this subject at length.

Sudden hormonal change

In women, menstruation, pregnancy, and menopause can all result in a dramatic alteration in the threshold for headache. The various inputs here have been discussed in Chapter 2.

Change in barometric pressure

In Chapter 1, thunderstorms were included on the long list of factors that Cindy McCain identified as causing her headaches. This complaint is not uncommon in headache and migraine sufferers, and I have seen it in both directions: some headaches begin when a storm occurs, and other headaches are relieved once the storm breaks. Thunderstorms are a significant contributor to the naturally occurring electromagnetic radiation (EMR) we experience, discussed shortly. A simple way of viewing this is as a sensitivity to change in barometric pressure.

Medication dependence or withdrawal

Medication dependence and withdrawal are overlooked aspects of recurring headaches. Patients often identify something else. Some will say, 'Oh, but in my case it's just chocolate that causes my headaches' or 'It's just perfume.' I would disagree. If it were as simple as this, they would be avoiding that item and would not be seeing me. If they are still getting symptoms, it may be because they understand and avoid the triggers, but are still loading bullets into the gun. Routine medications can become one such 'bullet'. I need to help them understand that unloaded guns don't go off all by themselves.

In considering causes, remember Marjorie, who sat so miserably retching in my waiting room. The only things we ever really identified as problems for her were ergot medication and green food colouring. In this regard, you might say that Marjorie's case was unusual. In contrast, Iris's headaches seemed to require several interventions, and one of these was clearly to remove the prescription medication.

SOME UNUSUAL CAUSES OF HEADACHE

The means by which we can classify a headache is one of themes of this book. Are they defined by their frequency, the degree of disability they cause, their genetic associations, or the drugs to which they respond?

Another way of looking at them is the curious fact that some are characterised by one outstanding feature, and this feature is what they are named for. Let us look at some of these.

Cheese

We discussed the various dietary causes of headaches in the last chapter. As we have seen, some people do not link their headaches to food at all, and some people feel that a link exists but cannot nail the culprit. There is another group who experience a clear association. Besides red wine and chocolate (usually dark chocolate), cheese is one of the foods most commonly cited. This is not surprising when we consider the number of reactive ingredients in cheese (see Chapters 6 and 12 for more information).

Cough

As the name implies, these headaches occur when the patient coughs or causes straining around the head and neck in some similar manner. Cough headache is sometimes reported by migraineurs. The Mayo Clinic divides cough headache into two types.

- Primary cough headaches: usually benign in nature, they are probably the result of an increase in intracranial pressure.
- Secondary cough headaches: these have some other underlying cause, including the shape of the skull, or the presence of a brain tumour or an unusual collection of defects known as Chiari malformations.

Modern imaging techniques can help to clarify the more serious of these headaches.

Crying

Although crying is not often discussed as a trigger, many migraine patients and sufferers of tension headache report that serious crying can end in a headache.[57] Stress, hormonal effects, and muscle tension around the head and neck have all been offered as explanations. Even dehydration has been suggested as a cause. Whatever the correct answer may be — and possibly all of these contribute — it is certainly a common experience, judging from the patient stories I hear.

Electromagnetic radiation

We can widen the discussion on headaches caused by changes in barometric pressure to include the theory that the fields generated by electromagnetic radiation can trigger headache, depression, chronic fatigue, or sick-building syndrome.

If diet has been controversial as a theory in headaches, it is overtaken by debates about electromagnetic radiation. Once again, the controversy is fuelled by the fact that some people seem to be totally unaffected.

Let us unpick this one.

Electrical and magnetic fields are an integral part of the natural physical world around us. These fields mostly originate from the sun, and from thunderstorms. The nature of this kind of radiation is known as 'non-ionising', as opposed to the ionising radiation that we get from an X-ray. So although the frequency is too low to ionise, or split an electron off an atom, this radiation can still impact the making and breaking of delicate chemical bonds. One of the known effects of this is heating of affected tissues. Many people who feel that they are EMR-sensitive often comment on a warm sensation around the ear when using a mobile or cordless phone. The EMR comes from the charged particles (predominantly electrons and protons) of what scientists refer to as 'matter'.

Such fields exist in our bodies, from the electrochemistry of our cells through to electrical conduction within our muscles and nerves. Neurologists utilise this fact when they test you with an EEG or a nerve conduction study. Your doctor uses their activity to take an ECG reading of your heart.

Yet into modern life has come a major new player: artificially generated electromagnetic radiation, the result of domestic electrical installations. Once this might have been the light globe hanging from the ceiling, but we now live in a smog of radiation. Mobile phones, microwave ovens, computer screens, intercoms, and electric clocks are just some of them. In addition, some people are exposed because of nearby high-voltage power lines. Those whose bedheads are next to a power box on the outside wall get an extra dose. Many suspect that using a cordless phone increases your risk of headache. A landline-connected phone is much safer.

A lot of controversy has arisen recently, as some people living near wind farms have complained of a range of illnesses, which include headache and autoimmune disease. While the current official position in most countries seems to be that wind farms exert no negative health effects at all, several possibilities have been recognised. For example, the flicker frequency might affect people with photosensitive epilepsy (and migraine?), and the Australian National Health and Medical Research Council recommends that the flicker frequency remains below 2.5 hertz.[58]

Other possible concerns regarding wind farms include 'infrasound' (generally dismissed on the grounds of 'no evidence'), the alteration of barometric pressure in the vicinity of the turbines, and the generation of EMR fields nearby.

This is not the place to go into claim and counterclaim regarding wind farms. We will look at just a couple of possible mechanisms whereby factors such as EMR may affect health.

First, we start with melatonin. We saw on pages 96–97 that light turns off the production of melatonin. It is the magnetic field of light that does this. If electromagnetic radiation has the capacity to reduce our melatonin production, as has been suggested, it is a serious health risk indeed, and headache should come as no surprise.

Another possible mechanism is this: most doctors, quite early on in medical school, learn about a mysterious concept known as the blood–brain barrier. Or at least, I found it mystifying, and perhaps less was known about it in those days, before the widespread use of electron microscopes in medical research. What we knew was that certain bacteria, toxins, and even drugs could not get into the brain from the circulation because of this barrier. Now we know that the surface of the tiny brain capillaries has cells that join together to create 'tight junctions'. Cells such as microglia and astrocytes acts as sentries, deciding what can get in and what can get out. We discuss the role of these special cells in Part III of this book. What matters here is that dysfunction of the blood–brain barrier has been linked to the development of Alzheimer's and Parkinson's disease. Peptides (from food and neurotransmitters) can cross the blood–brain barrier;

chemicals, such as aspartame (an artificial sweetener), can do likewise. We also know that the blood–brain barrier works hard to shift glutamate out of the brain, maintaining a healthy balancing act.

As we can see, the barrier defence of the blood–brain barrier is a delicate thing at best. It was not 'designed' to resist some modern chemicals such as aspartame, which get across it anyway. It is 'designed' to control glutamate levels, but did not expect high-additive loads of MSG.

So the really scary thing that we are now learning is that EMR can affect the permeability of the blood–brain barrier. Extensive research has been carried out to this effect: from the CSIRO in Australia, to research facilities in Sweden, to Boston University, to the World Health Organization. If this needs to be spelt out further, what is being demonstrated is that a more leaky (or even more closed-up) blood–brain barrier, caused by EMR, is affecting the defences of our most important organ. In a world with more environmental and dietary toxins, nature's best way of warning us that something is seriously wrong may be to give us a headache.

Friday nights

The so-called 'Friday-night headache' comes on at the end of the working week. It is often associated with migraine, but not exclusively so. The theory is that the sufferer carries stress throughout the week, but stress hormones keep a clamp on the arteries of the scalp. Once the weekend comes and the person relaxes, the clamp comes off, and the throbbing and pain begin. It may seem counterintuitive that relaxation should have this effect, but it is a frequently reported trigger.

Some patients even report that the first few days of their holidays have been marred by headache. It would seem that this is more likely to be true of shorter breaks, such as a weekend break, or brief relaxation sessions.

Here we need to make the distinction between good and bad stress. It does seem that 'good' stress is actually beneficial, and relief from it is unlikely to lead to a headache. But 'bad' stress is usually defined as stress to which there seems to be no resolution. With 'bad' stress, we have brought our problems with us. The cortisol and adrenalin that kept us going are withdrawn, leading to the process just described.

Pleasant relief may come from yoga, a massage, or a holiday. These modalities may help us put our problems in perspective. However, caution must prevail. One patient I know went to a chiropractor, and the neck manipulation led to the worst migraine she had ever had. In fact, she was taken to hospital with a suspected stroke. I must say on record here that, although it is not an uncommon practice, I cannot recommend neck manipulation, as opposed to neck massage, for any form of headache.

Hats or goggles

Compression of the nerves — or, indeed, the blood vessels of the scalp — is probably the cause of this type of headache. Also called a 'compression headache' by the Mayo Clinic, it can be brought on by wearing tight swimming goggles, helmets, headbands, and hats. More common in migraine sufferers, it is thought to afflict about 4 per cent of the population.

Hot dogs

This term, 'hot-dog headache', has been applied to people who experience headache after eating not only hot dogs, but also ham, bacon, and other cured meat products. Often these are the only known precipitants. The reaction usually occurs within half an hour, and is often accompanied by facial flushing. It would seem that the culprit here is nitrite, which dilates blood vessels.

The unpredictability of this headache may be connected with ambient temperature, reflecting the difference between eating a hot dog in the hot sun at a fairground and eating one indoors on a cold day. For more on nitrites, see Chapter 12.

Ice-cream

If you want a 'scientific' name for this curious headache, it is *sphenopalatine ganglioneuralgia*. In plainspeak, when you put something very cold in your mouth, it stimulates the sphenopalatine nerve, which feeds into the trigeminal nerve and the trigeminal ganglia. For more on the role of the trigeminal ganglia in headaches, see Chapter 12.

Sometimes this headache is known as 'brain-freeze' headache. People who experience either facial flushing or headache when they are suddenly exposed to very cold weather are probably activating the same neural pathways as in the ice-cream headache. Eating ice-cream more slowly, or gradual exposure to cold weather, are good solutions.

The pain of an ice-cream headache usually peaks within 60 seconds and does not last more than about five minutes. Only persistent pain or other unusual symptoms would warrant seeking medical attention. The phenomenon is common enough to have been the subject of research published in the *British Medical Journal* and *Scientific American*.[59]

Sex

It is a longstanding joke that women wanting to avoid sex say, 'Not tonight, darling, I've got a headache.' We will not go into the sexual politics of this excuse, but sometimes the headache is real. As a migraineur, I know that during a headache or migraine aura, sex is the last thing on anyone's mind. It just so happens, as we have seen, that women outnumber men three to one in the migraine department. However, the number of men who experience this kind of headache is also quite significant.

The benign sexual headache

Sometimes a headache is brought on by sexual activity. This category is recognised by the US National Headache Foundation and the International Headache Society. Two kinds are usually described.

- In the first kind, sexual excitement and exertion lead to muscle contraction in the head and neck, tripping pain pathways.
- In the second kind, the headache is probably caused by a sudden surge in adrenalin that occurs just before orgasm. Exertion is not generally involved. The pain is typically severe, and the condition has been dubbed 'orgasmic headache' or 'orgasmic cephalalgia'. It is more common in men than women.

Both kinds of benign sexual headache are more common in migraine sufferers, and show some response to migraine medications.

Although sexual headaches are usually benign, pathology such as stroke and tumour could declare themselves in this manner.

Cluster headache
This is another category of headache that may be related to sex. It can be triggered by sexual activity, or even by sexual frustration. Cluster headaches, while not life-threatening, could hardly be described as 'benign'.

Headache relief
One patient asked me whether 'needing sex' could trigger a migraine. She has severe migraines and carries a double dose of the MTHFR mutation. She enjoys a good relationship with her husband, and sexual frustration is not an issue. However, she has commented that sometimes, when the headache has dragged into a second or third day, she finds that sex can act as a circuit-breaker. It turns out that she's not alone. For more on this topic, see Chapter 13.

Space
It is unlikely that many of us will ever get to experience a space headache, but some Dutch neurologists who studied 17 astronauts found that these very fit individuals suffered disabling headaches while in space. The researchers ruled out motion sickness as the cause, and blamed painful pressure on the brain secondary to increased blood flow. They conjectured

that the headaches resulted from the effect of zero gravity, leading to redistribution of blood flow in the upper body. [60]

This example would fit into the vascular theory of headaches, discussed in the next chapter.

Weather

'Weather headache' is another term for the changes in barometric pressure, which we have already discussed. Storms or wind are the most common precipitants. Our language reflects the significance of this: in English, we talk of an 'ill wind'; Germans call it *Föhn*; in the west of North America it's *chinook*, and in Israel it's *sharav*.

Scientists probably know more about the sensitivity to barometric pressure in birds than in humans. Birds are thought to be finely tuned to the variance of pressure between their internal cavities and the outside air. Humans have cavities such as the sinuses and the middle ear; we become aware of them during landing in a plane, or if suffering a sinus infection.

Yom Kippur

The 'Yom Kippur headache' or 'Ramadan headache' is the name for the head pain experienced by people who fast. Part of the cause could be caffeine withdrawal, as the faster abstains from tea and coffee, and many of the food-withdrawal reactions already discussed could be contributing.

When Muslims observe Ramadan, they sometimes experience symptoms during the first week or two of the holy month. The most common of these is headache, and low blood sugar is not thought to be the problem. Interestingly, such headaches seem to regress as the month proceeds, lending weight to the idea that withdrawal of reactive foods may be the cause.

While these unusual headaches have a curiosity value of their own, the terminology makes an important point. Sufferers often have a very clear idea of what provokes their headache, and they should be listened to. In my student days, it was not uncommon to hear more paternalistic doctors say, 'Oh, such and such food/activity doesn't cause headaches; you're wrong.' Luckily, that is all changing.

CHAPTER 5
Psychology and Pain: what's happening in my head?

'Traditional cultures and technological civilisation start from opposite assumptions. In every traditional culture the psychotherapy, belief systems, and drugs needed to withstand most pain are built into everyday behaviour and reflect the conviction that life is harsh and death inevitable. In twentieth-century dystopia, the necessity to bear painful reality ... is interpreted as a failure of the socioeconomic system ... Pain thus turns into a demand for more drugs, hospitals, medical services ...'
IVAN ILLICH, *LIMITS TO MEDICINE*

If ever anyone was cynical about the limits of modern medicine, it was the philosopher, priest, and linguist Ivan Illich. His 1971 book *Deschooling Society*, which analysed modern institutionalised education, first brought him to public attention, and he followed it with *Limits to Medicine* in 1975. We might imagine that he would be aghast at the plethora of drugs now created to relieve pain that may arise from environmental insults of our own making, and from medical schooling that is propped up by the manufacturers of those drugs.

But let us take a closer look at that pain. Should we re-examine it to enable some better solutions? Does the 'gun, bullet, trigger' approach help us?

In a move that could incense the severe headache sufferer, researcher Peter Goadsby set out to explore the possibility that the pain experienced during a migraine may be an illusion.[61]

The idea is not entirely ridiculous.

It is easy to find situations that illustrate how the mind mediates the perception of pain. Eating chilli makes you feel as if the lining of your mouth is being blowtorched — but not much is actually happening to the cells that form that lining. A bird that eats a chilli (studies have been done on chickens) doesn't feel any burning sensation at all.

You probably know that any pain feels worse when you are tired and hungry. During a migraine, skin sensations, lights, and sounds that you can normally tolerate may become unbearable. The skin sensations are called 'allodynia' or 'hyperalgesia'; in the case of light and sound, it's 'photophobia' and 'hyperacusia' respectively. In contrast, nitrous oxide (not to be confused with nitric oxide), known as 'laughing gas', will make a child giggle while a doctor completes a painful procedure. Asked if it is hurting, the child will smile and nod, and then burst into peals of laughter because they are dissociated from the pain they are still feeling. So perhaps it is not impossible that the headache victim's pain is 'all in the mind'.

WHAT IS HEADACHE PAIN?

If it were a dog, you'd shoot it. What is happening in my head?

To understand headache pain, we need to look at some anatomy and chemistry, which is introduced below and discussed in detail in Part III of this book. Here we can briefly say that the trigeminal nerve (see Chapter 11) seems to be implicated in the pain pathways of *all* headaches. Take a look at Diagram 2.

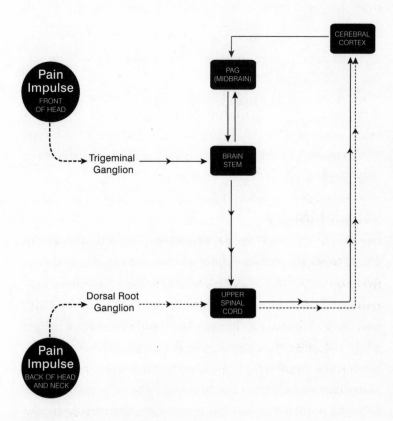

Diagram 2: pain pathways

Goadsby developed his ideas on the mechanisms of migraine in 2003, but his comments are no less interesting now than they were then. His theory begins with the fact that the brain itself has no pain-sensing neurons; therefore, the pain must be experienced in the meninges, the membranes that cover the brain. The big question is how the pain gets started, and there are three theories.

- The vascular theory: it originates when the blood vessels that supply the meninges dilate, leading to throbbing.
- The neuronal theory: it originates in the delicate neurones of the trigeminal nerve that supply those blood vessels.
- It is created by inflammation triggered by messenger molecules.

Let us look at the first two in detail, before we look at the third possibility.

Vascular theory

Because more has been written about migraine than most other headaches combined, let us start there. For a long time it was thought that the pain of migraine had a vascular origin. After all, the brain itself is relatively insensitive to pain. Indeed, neurosurgeons can cut into brain tissue with a scalpel while the patient is awake, but little or no distress is felt. Electrical stimulation on the cerebral cortex may produce no more than a tingling on the opposite side of the body. Pain is part of a warning system, and generally damage to tissues creates pain, but Mother Nature did not anticipate the effects of modern neurosurgery on the brain. In the distant past, by the time your brain was being cut, it was all over anyway. So it was easy to assume that the pain must be coming from the blood vessels.

Among the things we *do* interpret as a threat are injury, inflammation, and infection anywhere in the head and neck. With these assaults, blood vessels within the skull or on the face and scalp might dilate and throb, so the vascular theory of pain has relevance for more than just migraine.

Another thread of the vascular theory of headache pain relates to platelet aggregation (see Chapter 2). If platelets aggregate to form a tiny clot in tiny blood vessels, blood supply in that area would be reduced. The person may have a small clot (which could lead to a mini-stroke). Larger blood vessels may even be involved and produce a full stroke, as can happen with familial hemiplegic migraine. Pain could result as a signal that something is wrong. A recent study showed that from 1995 to 2008, the rate of stroke in women aged 20 to 44 doubled.[62] The possible relevance of this will be discussed in Chapter 7.

Neuronal theory

Mother Nature needs to deploy other warning systems, and so she sends signals by fibres that interpret pain. These, of course, are our nerves. They may be activated by stimuli ranging from injury and inflammation through to a rise in pressure within the skull or in the sinuses. Sinuses are those cavities within the bones of the skull. With a bad sinus infection, the mucosal membranes that line them come under pressure, and we feel a full sensation that can cause throbbing pain. If there is an abscess or a haemorrhage in the brain, the meninges get stretched, and we know that something is amiss. In these cases, the pain message is clear.

But sometimes the pain seems out of all proportion to any perceived threat or damage. In these cases, headache researchers use the term 'neuronal dysfunction'. This occurs when the pain messages get scrambled, or one message triggers another and they spread like a bushfire. Neuronal dysfunction occurs when a simple warning signal gets exaggerated by a positive feedback loop.

Let me give you a couple of examples. A bright light or glare may warn of damage to our eyes. A concussive blow should tell us to take evasive action. But is there any value when a bright light causes you to nurse a headache for hours or days, or a bump on the head puts you in hospital with anaphylaxis? The first scenario is not uncommon for migraine sufferers. The second is a rare but interesting occurrence. In the emergency room, I once saw a patient brought in in a state of collapse with an unusual condition known as 'hereditary angioedema'; a mild bump on the head had put her into anaphylactic shock. Some people have a similar response to sudden cold; the symptoms may range from hives (called 'cold urticaria') to anaphylaxis. More common forms of anaphylaxis can be seen as the body's same overshoot response.

Inflammatory messenger molecules

Closely linked to neuronal dysfunction is the third major theory of headache pain. According to this theory, a messenger molecule, such as a cytokine, sets off a biochemical cascade that activates pain signals and overrides the normal mechanisms that control pain.

Of course, these separate theories are arbitrary; they are no more useful than any other chicken-and-egg discussion. Nerves communicate their messages by means of neurotransmitter molecules. Every part of our body is directly or indirectly in dialogue with almost every other part. Comparison can be made to our modern communications systems, which range from snail mail via air, road, or rail to email via satellite, telephone, or wireless network. The message may travel a long distance, or go to someone in the next room.

The body's messenger system is similarly varied, involving messenger molecules such as hormones, neurotransmitters, and cytokines. Some act locally, and some travel in the bloodstream and act on the receptor sites of distant cells. Others use the electrical circuitry of the nervous system to send the message to a distant location. Both nerve impulses and messenger molecules affect organs such as the adrenal gland, muscles such as the heart, and blood vessels in various locations.

WHERE DOES THIS FIT IN WITH HEADACHES?

Where headaches are concerned, a busy conversation takes place within our body. It involves the muscles in the neck; sensitive surface structures, such as the teeth or eyes; balance organs in the inner ear; and the various pain centres in the brain. Rather than a simple dialogue between two parties, it is akin to question time in parliament. Everyone wants to have their say, and images of the tower of Babel are hard to suppress. The conversation may become an argument, but it's hard to say who started it. Perhaps the trigger was one provocative statement that brought up underlying tensions and memories, so that you can't easily apportion blame. So much for theories of causation where pain is concerned.

The work of Goadsby and others led him to believe that branches of the trigeminal nerve take their messages to the brainstem; from there, messages go to the blood vessels, instructing them to dilate. He argues that the sensory *input* into the trigeminal nerve is no more painful than it would be in any non-headache sufferer. It is the brainstem's *processing* of those messages that results in the overreaction that is experienced as headache (the neuronal theory). The idea is that the messages heading out of the brainstem go to the rest of the brain, and then loop back to the brainstem, where a dampening down of the pain signal should occur. If it does not, a positive feedback loop of pain is triggered, leading to the release of neuropeptides, neurotransmitters, other neuromodulators — and to headache.

One of these neurotransmitters is glutamate, and in Chapter 2 we saw the genetic reasons for the difficulty that some individuals have in clearing glutamate. There we also saw how the release of potassium ions and glutamate was part of the pain experience of headache. The genetics of abnormal glutamate and potassium chemistry were introduced in Chapter 3, and the story of the chemical outcome is continued in Chapters 12 and 13. The role of glutamate and the blood–brain barrier, discussed elsewhere, is also relevant in this context.

Furthermore, we know that people with serious mutations in the genes for calcium and sodium pumps have an increased risk of various headaches. Part of the action of these ion pumps is to modulate the messages the nerves are sending. The theory that pain is an illusion caused by a simple failure to switch off a chemical message is deflating, but I find it attractive. It helps explain why breaking any part of the circuit can make a difference. In terms of the gun image, it does not matter whether you remove the bullets or inactivate the trigger — you still gain some control over the headache. The theory also serves to explain how some determined individuals manage to control their headaches through meditation, yoga, massage, or similar techniques. And finally, if we go back to Illich's words and think of traditional cultures lacking the dubious 'luxury' of pharmabusiness, can we imagine that products such as monosodium glutamate would permeate the food supply if it was known to make even one person ill?

Circuit-breakers

When I said that I was writing a book on headache, a colleague remarked that if she wrote a book on headaches, it would be very short. She dispatches all her headache patients to the physiotherapists, and 'they all get better'. I reacted with cynicism. After all, I was seeing people who had been to specialist migraine clinics and were still suffering, people who 'did everything right' until we discovered that they were closet perfume addicts or had a specific food trigger.

As a child, I had personally experienced serious migraine when physically active and otherwise very healthy. At the time, I rode horses, studied classical ballet, and was soon to become a competitive swimmer. Surely I had no musculo-skeletal problems that would require a physiotherapist? Something else is at work here.

My colleague is a very competent and engaging doctor. Patients really *like* seeing her. They trust her. If she believes that physiotherapy is going to fix them, maybe it will. There is no shortage of evidence for placebo responses in headache or anything else. Perhaps that placebo response acts as a circuit-breaker, and thus stops the feedback loop of pain. Physiotherapy helps stretch and relax tight muscles, tendons, and ligaments.

Disciplines such as physiotherapy, chiropractic, and Pilates all have inputs into the sympathetic and para-sympathetic nervous systems. Most of the ancient healing arts involve physical therapies. Meditation and yoga are recognised as having neuromodulatory effects, even by hardline advocates of Western medicine. If they relieve your headache, do we label this 'psychological'? Perhaps we do, because neuroscience and the neurotransmitters are at the cutting edge of understanding illness and disease. The book *The Brain that Changes Itself* by Norman Doidge has enormous popular appeal, and not just among lay readers. Doctors from all backgrounds endorse it with enthusiasm.

The psychology of headache is one of the condition's most fascinating aspects. It has to do with that most elusive thing, 'human nature'. This covers the whole range of factors. Why is it that some people survive terrible life events, such as war, displacement, bereavement, serious illness, and loss, and despite all the odds, emerge as resilient optimists? Why is it that others lead relatively sheltered lives and yet still find the world a threatening place?

WHAT IS KNOWN ABOUT PAIN?

The exploration of these questions goes beyond the scope of this book. All we can say is that every one of us is a unique constellation of nature and nurture, a combination of our genetics and our life experience in general. What we can do here is explore a few of the 'knowns' about pain.

The expectation of pain

When I was a young doctor working on a surgical ward, the anaesthetist in charge was a wise older man with a straightforward approach to pain: 'Never let the patient learn to expect pain.' This was in contrast to the rule of the day (applying still in some places) that opiate analgesia should be given only once in four hours. But this doctor believed that if you relieved pain early, the patient would be off analgesia altogether much more quickly.

He was ahead of his time — subsequent years have shown that patients who can self-administer pain relief use much less analgesia in total than those who lie watching the clock waiting for their next budgeted respite.

The brain learns about pain

It has now become apparent that people who put up with headache pain often become harder to treat in the long run.

Those who have learned that headache is a debilitating illness live in fear of it. When patients no longer expect regular headaches, they sometimes experience relief even when the bullets and triggers remain. They find that they do not have headaches at all, or that their headaches are less frequent and easier to manage than previously. This relief may be due to the interventions themselves. But it would seem that being free of the fear of headaches they cannot control also plays a role.

The pharmacology of pain

It is now well recognised that overuse of medications can lead to headaches when the drugs are withdrawn. This is one reason that some doctors are cautious with pain relief. The pain of withdrawal is not a psychological consideration; it is a true drug effect. But doctors are also keen to get adequate headache control because of the factors we have just been discussing. They recognise that once the brain has learned the pain response, it is likely to activate — and, indeed, escalate — this response.

Thus far I am in agreement with the conventional wisdom. But we need to take a step back. Few people would think of their headaches as an analgesic deficiency. If the root cause of the headache is sensitivity to perfume or food, it is a no-brainer to address these basic problems before we use a drug to fix the symptoms. I find it very difficult and frustrating to try to address the iatrogenic (doctor-caused) problem at the same time as dealing with the environmental and genetic ones.

The psychology of pain

Most of the children in the Great Ormond Street study (Chapter 3) were described as exhibiting behavioural disturbances at the times of the attacks. This is hardly surprising. Children are not always articulate in describing something as straightforward as 'pain'. An adult who tries describing what 'dysphoria', 'panic', or even 'depression' feels like will get the picture. A child plays up when it feels bad.

Now that science is teaching us more about the chemistry of emotions such as panic or depression, and the effects of serotonin and other neurotransmitters, we realise that it is academic whether the pain causes the anxiety, the anxiety causes the pain, or a chemical reaction gives rise to both at the same time. It was notable in the Great Ormond Street study that when the headaches were controlled, the improvement in behaviour was dramatic. Some years after the study was done, I had the privilege of meeting one of the paediatric psychiatrists who had worked with the children. She confided that the outcomes went beyond her most optimistic expectations, to the point that she wondered what role diet was playing in much of the psychiatric illness she saw.

One of the behaviours in question was hyperkinetic activity in everyday life (about half the children), and other symptoms described as 'illness-behaviour', observed during the attacks. These kids were happier when on the appropriate diets.

But are we surprised? MSG is one of the factors that ramp up the balance of excitatory glutamate. Mild excitement can be fun; too much leads to irritability and disruptive behaviour.

Food colourings send rats crazy when they are exposed to fluorescent lights. Why not kids?

What can we learn from complex regional pain syndrome?

Chapter 13 discusses nociceptive (pain) receptors in some detail, but the link to headache was introduced in Chapter 1. There I mentioned the work of Professor Martin Pall, and his idea that our (genetically influenced) NMDA receptors are key players. Under the ambitious title *Explaining Unexplained Illnesses*, he makes a cogent case that environmental chemicals lead to neural sensitisation. This, he says, happens when enzymes are stimulated by these chemicals to produce nitric oxide. That then leads to the inappropriate release of glutamate.

In simple terms, this means the brain learns about pain, comes to expect it, and can be sensitised to it. Some of us are more genetically at risk of such problems.

In CRPS, the key complaint is pain, but the skin of the affected area develops hyperalgesia (an exaggerated response to pain or touch). Both migraine and chronic tension headache can be accompanied by hyperalgesia. In Martin Pall's terms, CRPS, chronic fatigue syndrome, and multiple chemical sensitivity are 'unexplained illnesses'.

Many headache sufferers express bewilderment and seek explanations for the frequency and severity of their headaches. They get weird symptoms, such as hyperalgesia or sensitivity to light and sound. They seem to hurt all over, react to everything, and feel pretty stressed and unhappy in the process.

The gut connection

We looked at a link between headache and the gut in Chapter 1, where I discussed the problem of irritable bowel syndrome, and also in Chapter 3, which looked at some immunology.

There is now an increasing awareness of the contribution of the gut and gut bacteria to the health of an individual. It is said that up to 80 per cent of our immune system resides in the gut; estimates vary, and some exceed that number. A large part of this gut-related immune system is made up of the teeming mass of bacteria in our gut, referred to as the gastrointestinal microbiome. It is my belief that future textbooks of immunology and medicine will have many chapters dedicated to the topic. It is worth a book in its own right, but here I want to recount the story of one study that seems relevant.

In this study, mice suffering from infectious colitis displayed anxiety behaviour. Anxiety plays a key role both in triggering headache and in worsening the pain of it. When the mice were treated with an important gut bacterium, *Bifidobacterium longum*, they became calmer. However, if the mice had undergone severance of the vagus nerve, the calming effect was not present.[63] The hypothesis is that healthy gut bacteria were able to facilitate the production of neurotransmitters such as serotonin. Indeed, it is thought that the gut microbiome is responsible for more than 90 per cent of our *entire body supply* of serotonin. As we trawl through the number of medications used to treat headaches and see how many of them target serotonin production, it is easy to see why this aspect of our biology is attracting increasing attention.

Chapter 12 takes this story a little further.

And to be the devil's advocate ...

Investigators at Bristol University have revisited a theory held by many doctors in the 19th century: that pain is an essential part of the healing process. Professor Paolo Madeddu led a study purporting to show that pain experienced during a heart attack marshals stem-cell repair and increases the chance of survival.[64]

Furthermore, Doctor Holly Strausbaugh, writing in *Nature Medicine*, argued that in joint disease the activation of pain pathways turned down the inflammatory cycle and stopped the inflammation from going into overdrive.[65]

How such research will play out for headache sufferers, I cannot say. I do have several patients who, despite long headache histories, have stoically resisted using medication, and they do not seem any worse off than those who have used a lot. Indeed, in attacking the causes of their headaches, we never have to deal with the complicating issue of drug dependence first.

Will Ivan Illich have the last word on this one after all, I wonder?

Politics and intrigue?

As we saw in Chapter 3, a 2007 *Lancet* report on food additives showed that children consuming benzoic acid derivatives and certain food colourings had an increased degree of hyperactivity when compared with controls.[66] But more than 30 years before this, the Great Ormond Street study had implicated these very food additives when observing behavioural responses in migrainous children. And more than 40 years before, in June 1973, Doctor Ben Feingold had presented similar findings before the annual conference of the American Medical Association. His list also included some foods high in natural salicylates, and synthetic colours, flavours, and preservatives (many of which are derived from petrochemicals). Could these chemicals that are connected with undesirable behaviour be contributing to headaches?

You have to wonder what forces keep such information from the public. Over the years, the medical profession has been on the front foot in deriding the Feingold Diet as useless. A quick search shows how the food industry itself can outmarket good science.[67] I would guess that many doctors in headache clinics remain uninformed about, and uninterested in, the food additives going into the mouths of their patients. And these are *sick* people, for whom a drastic regime of medication is often prescribed. It has taken four decades, and lots of derision, for Feingold's work to get the recognition it deserved from the outset. It has taken almost as long for the work done at Great Ormond Street, and by Doctor Jean Monro, on migraine in children, to be acknowledged. How many more decades will it take for adult migraineurs to routinely receive the option of a dietary trial?

So let us go back to the question that heads this chapter: 'What's happening in my head?' When headache expert Doctor Ninan Mathew spoke to *Time* in 2002, he said, 'Any recurring headache that is debilitating enough to keep you away from work or the things you enjoy is probably a migraine.' Would he still say the same thing today, after ten years of genetic research? My feeling is that he would. But I place the emphasis on his use of the word 'probably'. The point he was making was not to waste time defining what kind of headache it is. He was saying, 'We might as well call it something — "migraine" is as good as anything else.' Many pain pathways are involved, and understanding these is more important than minute classification of different headaches.

Not alone

Many patients I see are made so miserable by their headache cycles that they feel isolated and depressed. Some have supportive partners, but many feel that those around them are tired of their chronic ill health. The workplace can provide a challenge, especially knowing that others will have to cover their absence. This consideration alone can lead to early retirement.

A surprising number report that their neurologist has told them that they are the worst case the doctor has ever seen. One neurologist actually added, 'After myself, that is.' Can this really be the case — or do the doctors feel obliged to say something other than simply 'you have a chronic problem, and all we can do is keep prescribing different drugs for you'?

I hope this book will go some way towards offering other options. The sheer size of the problem certainly warrants better solutions. Although some people will take no comfort in simply knowing they are in good company, others may find it heartening to reflect on the following.

I have already mentioned Cindy McCain several times. Another example is Charlotte Brontë; despite a sad end, there is little doubt about the contribution she made to literature. We regret her early death, but also acknowledge that life expectancy was shorter then. Even though headaches are debilitating, headache sufferers have achieved much.

Who else might we find on a list of high achievers? There are obvious difficulties in making a retrospective diagnosis. However, there is general agreement that Julius Caesar and Napoleon Bonaparte, opponents Ulysses S. Grant and Robert E. Lee, and Thomas Jefferson are among historic political figures who are thought to have been migraineurs.

Writers include Lewis Carroll, who is said to have found the inspiration for *Alice in Wonderland* in his migrainous auras. Emily Dickinson famously wrote more than one poem on the experience of migraine and headache. Virginia Woolf is said to have suffered frequent migraines while writing novels such as *Mrs Dalloway* and *To the Lighthouse*. Both are classics, and in my opinion the latter is a contender for one of the most beautiful books in the English language. The literary list includes George Eliot, who described her attacks in a journal, and George Bernard Shaw, whose vegetarianism was apparently an attempt to cure his migraines.

Artists likely include Picasso, whom we discussed briefly in Chapter 4. In addition, George Seurat, Vincent van Gogh, and Claude Monet are all on the list of suspected migraineurs. Musicians apparently include Tchaikovsky, Chopin, and possibly even Elvis Presley.

In a category we might call 'thinkers', we find Karl Marx, Immanuel Kant, and Blaise Pascal. Friedrich Nietzsche apparently suffered migraine at boarding school. Charles Darwin is thought to have inherited his migraine from his grandfather Erasmus Darwin, a physician who studied the vascular theory of migraine (see page 114). Sigmund Freud is another 'thinker' with the problem, though his self-prescribed treatment with cocaine may have been as much the cause as the cure.

Migraine and epilepsy can have overlapping symptoms, and sometimes, particularly in the past, diagnosis was confused. Julius Caesar and Vincent van Gogh share this diagnostic dilemma, with distinguished medical historians arguing for and against migraine and epilepsy. Shakespeare clearly represents Caesar as an epileptic: Brutus says of him 'He hath the falling sickness.' Historians also portray Caesar as suffering from headaches and depression, especially in the last year of his life. Shakespeare has Othello suffering from epilepsy, depression, and headaches.[68] These examples are telling, but we must acknowledge the difficulty of making a retrospective diagnosis.

Modern celebrities who have suffered migraine include Princess Margaret and Whoopi Goldberg. Indeed, it seems that to be on the A-list, migraine is almost a requirement. At least, it appears that creativity and headaches might be linked. The neurotransmitters involved might explain this, or it could be the effect of people finding a way to survive their suffering.

PART II
Treatment Options

CHAPTER 6
Finding the Problem Foods: diets for headache

'You can know the name of a bird in all the languages of the world, but when you're finished, you'll know absolutely nothing whatever about the bird. So let's look at the bird and see what it's doing — that's what counts. I learned very early the difference between knowing the name of something and knowing something.'
RICHARD FEYNMAN

If food plays a role in headaches, perhaps following a diet can cure them? In the analogy of the gun, this represents taking the bullets out. The trouble-causing foods discussed in Chapter 3 give us plenty of suggestions about foods to avoid. The main problem is choosing a diet that will suit our needs. How do we go about this?

Every headache sufferer has inherited a different genetic makeup, has been exposed to different foods and chemicals, and has had different life experiences. There is no one-size-fits-all diet to fix headaches. Depending on the combination of the 'headache genes' we inherit and these other factors, we will all react differently to different diets. Some people may need a combination of diets. But one important message from this book is this: I have seen more headache sufferers benefit from dietary manipulation than from any other single intervention. It has been through dietary change that many people have been able to give up or drastically reduce their medications. And it is through dietary intervention that the impressive study results mentioned in Chapter 3 were achieved. In that chapter, I laid the foundations for a dietary approach to headache. In this chapter, I give you tools for finding a suitable diet for yourself.

Although finding the right diet may sound impossibly difficult, I am impressed by how easily many patients manage to do it for themselves. Once food becomes the focus of attention, people often develop an instinct for what is making them ill. Others find the going hard and need help. Some may need expensive tests, such as those for IgG (mentioned in Chapter 3).

The foods that we have 'abused' — either as a culture or as individuals — are likely to be the ones that now make us ill. For example, adverse reactions to corn occur widely in the United States, where just about everything — bread, sugar, whisky — is made from corn. Interestingly, and by contrast, African and Chinese cuisines have traditionally used a lot of peanut products, but true peanut allergy (anaphylaxis) is rare in both countries.[69] Maybe they have almost 'bred out' their peanut-sensitive individuals. Maybe foetuses adapt in the womb because their mothers eat these foods on a daily basis.

Or maybe, as has recently been suggested, people in these cultures have learned ways of preparing these reactive foods so that adverse reactions are less likely to occur.

THE ELIMINATION DIET

The elimination diet can help you to identify any unusual pain triggers. Some people will want to try an elimination diet based on avoidance of specific foods, or on previous experiences of dietary exclusion. For those people, the food lists near the end of this chapter may be helpful.

Rules for undertaking the elimination diet

You need determination and focus to undertake an elimination diet. There is no point in doing it unless you are thorough. Here are some rules that will guide you to success.

Before you start

- A trial diet is best followed under medical supervision. A dietician or doctor experienced in the use of elimination diets is ideal.
- The trial period should be at least three to six weeks for any useful conclusions to be drawn.
- Plan ahead. Set aside a period when you will be able to spend time preparing your food. Go shopping to ensure that you have a supply of 'safe' foods available. Identify cafes and restaurants near you that can cater to specific food needs.

- Gradually withdraw tea, coffee, and energy drinks. Abrupt discontinuation of these can cause severe headaches and will disrupt the trial from the outset.

During the trial

- Do not wear or use any perfumes, fragranced cosmetics, or aftershave at any time.
- Do not smoke.
- Continue medications prescribed for serious medical conditions. Keep optional medications and painkillers to a minimum.
- Persevere through initial symptoms of withdrawal, which generally last about a week. Because of the drug-like effect of many foods, headaches may increase in intensity in the early phases of the diet.
- Balance the strictness of the diet with its tolerability. The stricter the diet, the faster the diagnostic clues will emerge.
- Follow the diet properly or don't bother. Half-followed diets are inconclusive and misleading. Just cutting down on a food — especially whole foods, such as milk, wheat, corn, chocolate, citrus, and egg — will tell you nothing. Later, *after* the reactive foods have been identified, you can experiment with 'how much' and 'how often'.
- Keep a diary of what you eat and when headaches occur.
- If complete elimination is impractical, you might have to settle for restriction and reduction. It is relatively easy to eliminate whole foods, but it is more difficult

to eliminate specific food *chemicals*, such as salicylates and amines. However, do exclude foods known to be high in certain chemicals (see below).

- Do not eat artificial sweeteners, colourings, flavour enhancers, or preservatives during an elimination diet. Read the labels and avoid E numbers (codes for substances that can be used as food additives).

- Remember that this diet is for diagnosis, not treatment. Some elimination diets are very restrictive and may result in nutritional deficiencies if they are carried on indefinitely. Failure to remember this is the most common cause of people giving up on dietary trials.

After the trial

- Once you notice significant improvement, you can regard the trial as ended and begin to reintroduce the potential culprit foods one at a time.

- Choose one of the eliminated foods and eat it several times a day for about three days. If there is no reaction after this time, that food is probably safe, and you can try the next new food. Any food that causes a reaction usually does so quickly because any tolerance for it has been lost during the withdrawal phase. So it is unlikely that you will have to wait a week for a reactive food to declare itself.

- Once you have identified a list of reactive foods, and you have found that avoiding them helps the headaches, feel free to experiment. Some people find that they can eat their reactive foods in small amounts, or in rotation. Or they can eat the food so long as they are not pre-menstrual or stressed, or the food is not taken with other reactive foods. Some people find that they are okay with the food in one form but not another — with cheese but not milk, milk but not cheese, A2 milk but not A1 milk, goat's milk but not cow's milk, and so on.

THE BASIC EXCLUSION DIET

For those who have never tried an elimination diet, the basic exclusion diet is a reasonable place to start. It is not for the faint-hearted. Even if it is followed strictly, it does not always 'work', because every individual is different — but it is a good starting point. Remember that it is not designed to be followed forever. It provides a baseline over a number of weeks: if you lose your headaches while on this diet, it's upward all the way as you slowly work out which foods you can tolerate.

First, read the rules about elimination diets, above. As recommended there, before starting the diet take about a week to wean yourself slowly off caffeine, including tea, coffee, drinking chocolate, and energy drinks.

Then remove from your diet:

- all dairy products from animals
- all cereals containing gluten
- all yeast, moulds, and yeast extracts
- certain vegetables that have been linked to headaches

(common culprits include corn, onions, and the nightshade family, including potatoes, eggplants, chillies, capsicum, and possibly brussels sprouts and cabbage)

- legumes, especially broad beans (fava beans), soy, and peanuts (some people may tolerate lentils and chickpeas)
- most fruits, especially tomatoes (including tomato sauce and tomato paste), bananas, citrus fruits, mangoes, apples, plums, and berries
- everything that has an E number
- foods with high salt content
- smoked fish, fish with dark flesh, shellfish
- cured meats such as salami, bacon, and ham
- alcohol, soft drinks, and juice in any form
- most cooking oils, including canola oil, peanut oil, and vegetable oil
- all types of nuts
- sugar and honey
- sesame seeds
- all types of spices.

This may leave you wondering what is left to eat! Based solely on the findings of elimination diet trials, permitted foods are:

- lamb, rabbit, turkey, venison, kangaroo, and game meat, cooked plainly, with no sauce
- white fish, cooked plainly, with no sauce
- vegetables such as spinach, lettuce, swede, turnip, carrot, parsnip, taro, and sweet potato; brussels sprouts

and cabbage are allowed if they do not provoke bowel symptoms or wind

- fruits such as pears (peeled), apricots, pomegranates, and paw-paw; Lady Finger (sugar) bananas are okay if they're not over-ripe
- grains such as rice, rice pasta, gluten-free rice bubbles, and rice flour, and starches such as sago and tapioca
- seeds, such as chia seeds, amaranth, and quinoa
- gluten-free flour and bread — those made from the permitted grains and seeds, but without yeast (ensure commercial products do not contain milk, eggs, or soy)
- oils such as sunflower oil, coconut oil, and olive oil
- herbal teas and filtered water.

Eating out

When you're out and about, it can be hard to find suitable food. Sometimes you can't eat to a regular timetable and you need a snack to tide you over, but convenience stores can be very inconvenient for those who insist on eating unprocessed food without additives. Find some portable foods that you can tolerate — rice crackers, sulphur-free dried fruit, or plain jerky — and keep a stash handy.

Eating out can be especially difficult if you have several trigger foods. Waiters and chefs may be thoughtful in suggesting alternatives, but sometimes you are just another problem in their busy day. If you are attending a wedding or a special dinner, make your requirements known when you accept the invitation, and confirm them with the staff as soon as you arrive at the venue.

Airline staff can sound helpful when you make your booking, but when it comes time to eat, you might find that your special meal has not made it onto the plane and the cabin staff deny all knowledge. On long-haul flights, confirm arrangements with the airline before each leg of the journey, and — when possible — carry some food of your own, just in case.

OTHER DIETS

Many people find following the basic exclusion diet surprisingly easy and effective once they are used to it. But others, either because of previous experience or alternative information, will want to try another approach. So I have also given an overview of some other diets; a visit to a bookstore or an internet search will undoubtedly turn up more. I only advise that once you have chosen a diet, give it a fair trial. Stick to what you have chosen, and follow the rules.

Some elements of the following diets can apply in all cases. For instance, it is wise to cut down on salt even if you are not following the low-salt diet. Removal of caffeine, colours, and additives is also recommended in all cases.

The low-salt diet
The name of this diet speaks for itself, and it should be part of every headache sufferer's trial regime. It is estimated that a primitive diet contained about 2 grams of sodium a day. That is why salt was a luxury, and in some cultures even a currency.

A healthy diet in a modern environment, which does not involve heavy work or salt loss from perspiration, should contain a *maximum* of 4 grams of salt a day. It is estimated that the modern Western diet contains closer to ten grams, sometimes even more. Some of us are okay on that diet, but others of us will get high blood pressure or headaches, or both. A lot of that is to do with the genetic throw of the dice.

The hunter-gatherer diet (paleolithic diet)

During the estimated 200,000 years since *Homo sapiens* first walked this planet, our diet was made up of what we could hunt and gather. It is only in the last 10,000 of those years that agriculture broadened our choices, giving us a diet based on grains and dairy products. And of course, it is only the last 100 years that have seen the large-scale industrialised production of processed foods.

We shall not spend time here discussing the pros and cons of these diets. Suffice to say that many people, including headache sufferers, have found health benefits from following a diet of the food that hunters and gatherers ate. Various examples can be found on the internet and in books on the subject. (See the further reading list near the end of this book.)

The rotation diet

A rotation diet is most useful after you have worked out which foods are making you sick. The theory behind the rotation diet is that humans never ate any food all year round; we ate what was in season. You might have a good feed of cherries for a few months of the year, but then not see cherries again until the next season came around. Or you killed a buffalo, and the whole tribe ate the meat until it was all gone. Your next chance would not be until the next migration of buffalo. In this way, it is argued, we got regular breaks from all of the foods we ate, preventing intolerances from developing. Nowadays, by contrast, we can get our favourite foods from the supermarket and eat them all year round.

On a rotation diet, you may choose to eat foods you find reactive once every four days. Or you may choose to eat foods that are in season locally, rather than out-of-season fruits and vegetables that have been flown in from around the world.

The rotation diet should not be confused with an elimination diet, which is used to determine which foods you are reacting to. Its value lies more in broadening your diet once you have determined what is making you unwell.

The blood-group diet

Blood-group diets are usually discussed in terms of the ABO and Rh (Rhesus) blood group systems, determined by our red blood cells.

This diet follows the theory that the original, out-of-Africa blood group was O Rh negative, and that the groups A, B, and Rh positive are modern mutations. To make things even more complicated, people can be divided into 'secretors' (80 per cent of the population) and 'non-secretors' (20 per cent of the population). People with O negative blood are said to possess a poorer tolerance for the products of agriculture. These people, it is argued, should be on diets high in meats and vegetables, avoid grains and dairy products, and be careful with legumes. In turn, other people are directed to follow diets suitable to their blood group, such as A or B (and possibly positive or negative). However, the distinction between positive and negative, and especially your secretory status, are thought to have a rather minimal impact on the diet right for your blood type.

However, the picture is complicated by the studies of evolutionary geneticists, who have found that our closest relatives, the chimpanzees, are most likely to be blood group A. It is argued that O may not be the original blood type.[70] When we look at transplantation of organs, it is the *white* cell blood types, known as the human lymphocystic antigens, or HLA types, that concern us. I suspect that tests of the HLA, or white cell, blood types (which are prohibitively expensive at present) may eventually tell us more about who should be eating what. The type of HLA genes we inherit have already been linked to the development of a wide range of illnesses, including coeliac disease, Hashimoto's and Graves' diseases (both thyroid diseases), autoimmune diabetes, lupus erythematosus, and certain kidney diseases.

Some patients have reported to me that following a blood-group diet (as defined by the red cell blood types) has helped their health or their headache patterns. I have not used this approach as a first response, but I would not discourage anyone who wanted to give it a try. Indeed, so many patients who were originally cynical about this diet have improved a range of medical conditions outside of headache by following it that I have gradually come to feel that it deserves more attention and study.

The casein-free diet

This diet is simple: do not consume milk products from any animals whatsoever. This means milk from goats, sheep, buffalo, and cows, and if you are in Tibet or Nepal, no yak products either. This includes milk, cream, cheese, yoghurt, low-fat and full-fat milks (homogenised or otherwise), casein, whey, or 'milk solids'. Often biscuits, snack foods, and margarine contain cheese powder or milk solids, so you need to read labels.

Some people think that lactose-free milk is okay, but it's not. Lactose-free milk has only the *milk sugar* removed. If you are reacting to milk with a headache, most likely it's the *milk protein* that is the problem. To be 'lactose intolerant' means that your gut does not produce the enzyme necessary to break down the milk sugar, which ferments and causes gas or diarrhoea. Lactose-free milk is useful if milk is giving you wind and diarrhoea, but it is quite separate from the problem of dairy protein intolerance.

Another distinction arises when people say that they are okay with A2 but not A1 milk. This refers to the protein casein, which can further classified into 'A1 beta casein' or 'A2 beta casein'. Just to make things difficult, casein is not the only protein in milk; other proteins, such as lactoglobulins, exist as well. It may be that these, rather than the casein, are causing a reaction.

Hence the advice: remove *all* dairy products from *all* animals for the trial period. It is a small investment to do without milk for a few weeks to see if it may help the headaches. Later on, you will be able to experiment. Some people are okay when dairy comes in the form of yoghurt or cheese, but not as milk. For others, it is the other way around.

But to clarify your reaction to it, it must *all* come out in the trial phase. I usually advise against using soy milk at this stage, but rice milk seems to be an acceptable substitute, and children tend to like its sweet, insipid flavour.

When it comes to children, a dairy-free diet will not stunt their growth, and certainly not in a matter of just weeks. Many children live quite healthily on long-term dairy-free diets.[71]

The gluten-free diet

This diet excludes any product made from wheat, rye, barley, or oats. The gluten in each of these cereals differs slightly, and in the previous sentence they are listed in the generally agreed descending order of reactivity. As such, some claim that oats are safe even for coeliac patients to eat. However, oats have certainly been implicated in the headaches of many people that I have seen. We cannot say whether this was due to the gluten in them, or to some other specific characteristic of the oats.

Similarly, some people seem to be more tolerant of the more ancient types of wheat, such as spelt and kamut. For the purpose of a gluten-free diet, *all* of these products are excluded.

The gluten-free, casein-free diet

Many elimination diets remove gluten and casein. Such diets have been used both in an attempt at diagnosis and for long-term management of ailments ranging from arthritis to autism spectrum disorders, migraines, Ménière's disease, and learning difficulties. In the studies mentioned in Chapter 3, many people reacted to dairy foods and to cereals containing gluten. They may be reacting to the whole food, or the effect may be the result of opiates or alkaloids (see 'The legume-free diet', on the next page).

The grain-free diet

The grain-free diet is much the same as a gluten-free diet, but takes out corn and rice as well. Amaranth, which has been cultivated for about 8000 years, and quinoa are increasingly popular gluten-free products. There is some debate as to whether they are grains or seeds, though I suspect that distinction is academic. They may be better tolerated than some other foods because the West has had less exposure and 'abuse' through overuse.

In essence, the grain-free diet is a variation on the hunter–gatherer diet, which is based on the principle that such cultivated cereals were rarely eaten because they occurred only in small pockets.

For those people who say that 'there is nothing left to eat' on a grain-free, dairy-free diet, it is salutary to consider that Australian Aboriginal peoples were gluten- and dairy-free (the only exception being human breast milk) for 60,000 years, until the advent of white settlers.

The legume-free diet

Legumes seem to be a problem for some people. Blood-group diets make much of who is able to tolerate legumes and who is not; certain classes of legumes are said to cause different reactions in different blood groups. Regardless of your blood group, if you get abdominal cramps and wind when eating legumes, you should avoid them when you are on an elimination diet.

Among the common members of the legume family are peas, beans, lentils, soy, and peanuts. Some of these can be eaten in their natural state. Others, such as soybeans and lentils, require preparation, such as soaking and cooking, to be palatable. Wattle seeds and Moreton Bay chestnut seeds were used by Australian Aboriginals as a food source only after extensive soaking and heating to remove toxins. So there are legumes and legumes.

Peanuts can be simply a nutritious snack or cause life-threatening anaphylactic reactions and non-life-threatening headaches, depending on who you are. The reactions may be due to the alkaloid content, the glutamate content, or an IgE or IgG reaction to the peanut protein itself.

Another aspect of legumes is that they tend to be high in natural chemicals called 'lectins'.

The lectin-free diet

Strictly speaking, it is not possible to have a lectin-free diet because almost all food contains these specialised proteins. The scientist Paul Ehrlich, regarded as the 'father of immunology', was able to show that dietary lectins are antigenic, meaning that they could provoke an antigen antibody response.[72] Purified lectins are used to determine ABO blood groups, and do provide some plausible links to diets based on blood-group types.

Although all foods have lectin properties, those thought to be the most problematic in causing an adverse food reaction include the following.

- Dairy. Interestingly, the milk from Daisy, the average family cow, is suspected of causing far fewer adverse food reactions than that from modern dairy cows, which are bred for the ability to produce large amounts of milk. There are several possible reasons. Genetically, Daisy was more likely to be an ancient breed, producing A2 rather than A1 milk. Her milk was not homogenised, and homogenisation has been shown to be linked to a whole spectrum of possible adverse health effects. And finally, Daisy ate grass, whereas modern cows may be grain-fed. We suspect that lectins from grains can pass into milk, whether it is human breast milk or animal milk. So the diet of the modern dairy cow may be as much the problem as the milk itself in creating adverse food reactions.
- Grains, especially wheat and wheat germ, but also oats, rye, barley, millet, and corn. Sadly, even grains often thought 'less reactive', such as quinoa, rice, and buckwheat, still have relatively high levels of lectins.
- Legumes, especially dried beans, red kidney beans, soy, and peanuts.
- Vegetables of the nightshade family, such as potato, tomato, eggplant, and capsicum.

The low-chemical diet

Many people with headaches have been put on diets low in natural food chemicals. The chemicals in question are usually salicylates, amines, natural glutamates, and phenols. The lists that follow shortly are helpful for those who want to reduce these chemicals in their diets. One friend has removed all seeds from her diet and says that this has been of benefit, both with her headaches and to her health in general. Her thinking was that Mother Nature puts her greatest concentration of chemicals into the seed — salicylates, amines, and so on — and this idea certainly has appeal. I would add that seeds are often very high in free glutamate.

The chemistry of these various food chemicals will be discussed in Chapter 12, where we will look at the implications for headache in removing these from your diet. It is also important to remember that the complexity of nature's molecules is such that neat categorisation is not always possible. One food — or one food chemical — may appear under more than one classification system.

Particularly helpful is *Friendly Food*, a book put out by the Allergy Unit at the Royal Prince Alfred Hospital in Sydney; another is Sue Dengate's *Failsafe Cookbook* (see the further reading list near the end of this book).

FOOD ADDITIVES

I have already expressed the view that certain additives, such as flavour enhancers and artificial sweeteners and colours, have little place in a healthy diet, headaches or no. It is true that they and preservatives may reduce food poisoning in the mass production of food and when a long shelf life is required. I think they have no role in the diet of a headache sufferer or the diet of a child with severe eczema, chronic abdominal pain, or any of the learning and behavioural difficulties classified as autism spectrum disorders. There is an argument that we should eat only food that can go bad, and eat it before it does. One could say food that will not support life forms, such as mould or insect larvae, can hardly support human life.

I have a well-stocked pantry, along with the abundance of fresh food we buy and grow. You would be hard-pressed to find any of these additives in my kitchen:

- artificial sweeteners: aspartame, saccharin, and sucralose
- artificial colours: E102, 107, 110, 122–29, 133, 142, 151,155, and 160b
- flavour enhancers, such as E621: monosodium glutamate (MSG).
- nitrates and nitrites
- preservatives E200–03, E210–313 (benzoates), E220–28 (sulphites), E249–52 (nitrates, nitrites), E280–83, and E310–21.
- salami, bologna, sausages, bacon, or hot dogs (see Chapter 3 for foods naturally high in nitrates).

Natural food chemicals

Not all the foods in the following boxes contain the same amount of food chemicals as one another. If you want to avoid these chemicals, it is best to consult internet lists to get some idea of relative quantities. For example, eggs have quite high levels of glutamate, but as only free glutamate is a problem, they are usually regarded as 'low' glutamate foods. And in terms of nuts, walnuts and macadamias have only half as much free glutamate as peanuts or almonds.

Lists of salicylate and amine foods, categorised into 'high', 'medium', and 'low', are readily available. The lists included here are given as a guide only.

Foods high in amines

The foods listed here contain high levels of amines. In addition, some foods contain large quantities of a specific amine, such as dopamine or histamine, and they are listed separately on the next page.

- anchovies
- avocados
- bananas
- beer
- broccoli
- broad beans (fava beans)
- cheeses (especially aged)
- chocolate
- dates
- eggplant
- fish
- fish roe
- grapes
- grapefruit
- hydrolysed vegetable protein (HVP)
- kiwifruit
- meats (especially aged)
- miso
- mushrooms
- offal
- olives
- oranges
- passionfruit
- pineapples
- raspberries
- sauerkraut
- sausages
- soy sauce
- spinach
- sultanas
- tangelos
- tempeh
- tomatoe
- yeast extracts

Foods high in alkaloids and opiates

Chapter 13 discusses foods that contain high levels of these drug-like chemicals. They can become addictive in the way that the related opiate drugs are addictive. The following foods are best avoided in an elimination diet.

- caffeine
- citrus fruits
- eggs
- tomatoes
- gluten (gluteomorphin)
- milk (caseomorphin)

Foods high in dopamine and dopaminergics

Foods that contain dopamine, or related compounds that have an effect like dopamine, are said to be 'dopaminergic'. They include Cavendish bananas, broad beans (fava beans), and Italian green beans.

Foods high in histamine and histidine

Some headaches are known as 'histamine headaches', and a low-histamine diet may be prescribed. Histamine headaches are discussed further in Chapters 10 and 12. Foods that contain high levels of histamine and histidine include aged cheeses and meats, beer, cabbage (pickled, sauerkraut), cooked ham, eggplant, fish, and mortadella.

Foods high in glutamate and glutamic acid

Glutamate, first discussed in Chapter 2, demonstrates that there can be no hard and fast rules about what is natural and what is not. Glutamate chemistry is explained in detail in Chapters 3 and 13. It is a natural chemical, but high concentrations in food can cause problems. Foods high in glutamate include the following.

- almonds
- beans
- beets/juice
- cabbage
- cashew nuts
- cheeses (all, especially parmesan)
- dairy products
- eggs
- hydrolysed vegetable protein
- fish
- kombu seaweed
- meats
- mushrooms
- MSG
- parsley
- peanuts
- pistachios
- sodium caseinate
- soy protein isolate
- soy sauce
- spinach
- tomatoes (especially ripe tomatoes and concentrates)
- wheat
- yeast extracts

Foods high in phenyl-ethyl amines

These foods include aged cheeses and chocolate. Foods that contain phenylalanine, from which the body makes phenyl-ethylamine, include beans, lentils, nuts, and seeds, as well as dietary supplements.

Foods high in phenols

Phenolic compounds are among some of nature's miracle molecules, because they are powerful anti-oxidants (see Chapter 12). However, they are listed here because some people react to them.

- apples (different types vary — for example, Braeburn has more than double the phenol content of Golden Delicious or Fuji)
- asparagus
- bananas
- beets
- blueberries
- broccoli
- capsicum
- cherries
- cranberries
- garlic
- grapes
- kidney beans
- mandarins
- oranges
- red onions
- peaches
- pears (different types vary; levels are lower than apples)
- pinto beans
- plums
- spinach
- strawberries
- tangerines

Foods high in phenolic amines

These foods include spinach, red wine, and yeast products. Foods that contain phenols are listed shortly. Some amine foods have a phenol structure, including lemons (Meyer cultivar), mandarins, meats (especially aged), oranges, and tangerines.

Foods high in tryptamine

These foods include aged cheeses, dairy, eggs, and soybeans.

Foods high in tyramine

These foods include the following.

- aged cheeses (exceptions include fresh cheeses such as such as ricotta, cream cheese, and Neufchâtel)
- anchovies
- avocados
- bananas
- Brazil nuts
- broad beans (fava beans)
- cabbage (pickled, sauerkraut)
- cactus fruit (prickly pear)
- caviar
- chicken liver
- coconuts
- eggplants
- green beans
- figs
- fish
- ham (cooked)
- meats (aged or processed)
- miso
- peanuts
- pickled herring
- pineapples
- plums (especially red)
- raspberries
- red wine (especially chianti/sangiovese)
- sausages (fermented)
- shrimp paste
- snow peas
- sour cream
- soy sauce
- tempeh
- teriyaki sauce
- tofu
- yeast products
- yoghurt

Foods high in salicylates

Foods with high levels of salicylates include the following.

- apricots
- blackberries
- blueberries
- boysenberries
- capsicums (green)
- champignons
- cherries
- chicory
- chillies (red)
- coffee
- corn
- cranberries
- cucumbers (canned)
- curry powder
- dill powder
- endive
- guava
- honey (content varies)
- liquorice
- loganberries
- macadamia nuts
- olives (green)
- oranges
- oregano
- paprika
- pineapples
- plums
- prunes
- radishes
- raisins, dates and currants
- raspberries
- cantaloupe (rockmelon)
- strawberries
- sultanas
- tea
- thyme
- tomatoes
- turmeric
- water chestnuts
- watercress
- youngberries
- zucchinis
- aniseed powder
- canella powder
- cayenne pepper
- celery powder
- cinnamon powder
- *garam masala*
- mace powder
- mustard powder
- Worcestershire sauce

Foods high in methylxanthines
Methylxanthines are another subset of the plant family that contains alkaloids and opioids.

- cocoa and chocolate
- coffee
- cola
- guarana
- ilex (yerba mate)
- tea

Foods high in serotonin
These foods include aged cheeses, bananas, chocolate, dates, kiwifruit, mushrooms, pawpaw, pineapples, tomatoes, and walnuts.

When we look at these many lists of possible culprits, it can all seem overwhelming. That's why a diet that removes all food additives and common culprit foods, as described in the basic exclusion diet, may be easier than picking out particular foods. No one need ever be hungry on this diet; you can eat the safe foods in sufficient quantities to satisfy hunger.

David's story

We first met David in Chapter 1, when we were looking at the ways in which headaches impact on the lives of people who get them.

David was resistant to the idea of an elimination diet. He had read the literature on cluster headaches and was already avoiding alcohol, chocolate, bananas, and preserved meats. I felt that we couldn't make much progress without an elimination diet, so I suggested he return at a future date if he wanted to try a more restrictive approach.

About a year later he came back, and his arrival is etched in my mind. His appointment coincided with a severe headache. He wanted a room where he could lie down in the dark. He was feeling nauseous, and to me it seemed like a migraine. He didn't want any pain relief, and, almost bizarrely, said all that he wanted to do was to discuss trialling an elimination diet.

I refrained from commenting that I thought this kind of obsessive determination might be part of the pathology.

I still remember standing in the darkened room, explaining the rules for an elimination diet. He was acutely intolerant to sound, and so I had to speak quietly and stand quite near the head of the bed. This time, I also smelled his aftershave, which we discussed.

David began taking magnesium, and I saw him a few months later. He had successfully completed a trial diet. Such diets are hard to interpret when patients are not getting headaches regularly. Would it have been a headache-free period anyway, or was it the diet? David was convinced that the elimination of dairy products and wheat had made the difference. He now found all perfumes and air fresheners offensive, and avoided them.

A couple of years went by, and his wife came to see me on another matter. She reported that David was now completely headache-free.

I will probably never know what the true diagnosis was, and somehow it does not seem all that important.

CHAPTER 7
Avoiding Harmful Chemicals: perfume, cigarette smoke, and cleaning agents

'O Rose thou art sick.
The invisible worm
That flies in the night …
Does thy life destroy.'
WILLIAM BLAKE

Mary was one of my early migraine successes. She originally came to see me with a severe mood disorder and a worsening migraine, which had begun within days of her 40th birthday. Blood tests did not indicate menopause, but her detailed history gave us a clue. Discussing her birthday celebration, she commented that someone had given her an extremely expensive bottle of perfume. Yes, she always wore perfume: 'Doesn't every woman?' She had never worn this brand before. Yes, she had a migraine history, but the headaches were 'menstrual' and clearly (she said) had nothing to do with perfume.

The clue was that the surgeon Mary worked with — she was a nurse in the local hospital — had recently complained of a horrible smell and wondered if there was some vomit somewhere in the ward that had not been cleaned up. He noticed that the smell was stronger when he was near Mary, and she worked out that her new 'fragrance' was the culprit when the surgeon asked her to check her shoes. (I had always wondered whether there was something wrong with my sense of smell, but I learned from Mary that at least one surgeon shared my judgement.)

Firstly, Mary stopped wearing that perfume to work. Then, with my encouragement, she stopped wearing perfume altogether, and she washed her clothes and aired them. That was all. No dietary changes, no supplements.

The next time I saw her, the mood swings had gone, and so had the migraine. It sounds too easy, but sometimes it is just that simple.

In Chapter 4, I said that petrochemicals, perfume, and cigarette smoke were such potent triggers of headaches that they deserved a chapter of their own. Mary's story illustrates the significance of such triggers well, so let us delve into the issue more deeply.

OUR SENSE OF SMELL

We humans do not always rate the sense of smell highly. Compared with our ability to hear and see, it comes in at a poor third. There have even been suggestions that when we learned to live with dogs thousands of years ago, we relegated some of our ability to smell to our canine friends. Our ancestors, sleeping in caves and simple shelters, used dogs to alert them to threats. Although we talk about 'smelling danger', many of us rely on the family dog to guard the house and to guard us.

We can live without a sense of smell, but we are poorer for it. There are rare genetic disorders whereby some people are born without a functional olfactory nerve. I once knew such a person, who said that other members of her family were also afflicted. The only smell that she was aware of was water, and then only when the water was hot. It only takes a little imagination to work out why water might be the one odour detected by an undeveloped olfactory nerve.

We know that some people are born with a poor sense of smell, and that there are others whose sense of smell is acute. This is sometimes seen in conjunction with a heightened sense of sound, and indeed, children with autism spectrum disorders often experience both a heightened sense of smell and hyperacusis (inability to tolerate loud sounds). However, it is not just volume that these children are bothered by. They, along with many migraineurs, find certain other sounds unpleasant, or even deeply disturbing. For lovers of trivia, there is the truly bizarre story that no less than two musicians have died from heart attacks at exactly the same point while conducting Wagner's opera *Tristan and Isolde*. In what has become known as 'the curse of Tristan', the story becomes surreal because their deaths occurred at a place in the score where Wagner had used a musical interval known as the tritone. This is a chord with an augmented fourth, also called 'the devil's interval'. The musical representation of this interval was actually banned by the medieval Church, who clearly took the dissonance produced by a tritone very seriously.

But hyperacusis is only part of the full spectrum of sensory disorders; hypergnosia is another. This includes an aversion to certain smells and tastes. And people suffering from some mental illnesses, such as schizophrenia, often complain of bizarre smells. It is easy to dismiss this as paranoia, but we should weigh up the possibility that their sense of smell allows them to detect odours that the rest of us do not. The parallel here is with allodynia (pain caused by stimulus that doesn't usually cause pain), first introduced in Chapter 1.

Headache sufferers are more than usually sensitive to a range of sensory inputs. At the onset of a headache, many have a heightened awareness of sound, smell, and taste. Flickering and flashing lights and strobe lighting may be intolerable, and may precipitate a headache. This sensitivity is probably genetically based, and may be related to the inheritance of certain G-protein receptors (see Chapter 13).[73] During a headache, once certain nerves are switched on, the off switch doesn't seem to work very well.

Along with my history of migraines, I also have an acute sense of smell and taste. I have often found that I could re-create the ingredients in a curry without need of a recipe. If I had taken up oenology, I suspect I might have been successful. Although wine-tasting skills might not have been in nature's evolutionary brief, there are several potential benefits of an acute sense of smell.

Odour-induced nausea in pregnancy seems like a disadvantage, but current theory has it that nausea in pregnancy is protective to the foetus.[74] My patients with severe morning sickness are far more likely than average to suffer from headaches, particularly migraines. An acute and unpleasantly powerful reaction to strong odours is part of the extreme form of the condition *hyperemesis gravidarum*, but even milder forms see women eschew coffee, tea, or the use of toothpaste.

My acute sense of smell has enabled me to detect perfume on patients as we enter my office from the waiting room. They may protest that they have not applied any that day, but it often turns out that they are wearing clothes worn when they (or even a family member) was wearing perfume.

If we think of the potential value of this sensitivity in a bygone era, the odour-sensitive among us may have been the ones to detect leaks from a gas seam or the erupting volcano. We may have detected by smell that food was off and warned the rest of the tribe. It is only in modern times that this 'detector' has been defiled by a multitude of noxious smells. And maybe our headaches have been doing us a favour. The odours that we find offensive, as we will soon see, may be alerting us to carcinogens and other nasties in the chemical soup that surrounds us.

Our sense of smell may even help us to find a genetically suitable mate. Studies have shown that our ability to detect pheromones helps us to choose a partner who is not related to us, thus avoiding the perils of inbreeding. We read about the HLA haplotypes (also known as MHC genes) in Chapters 2 and 6. In research known as 'the sweaty T-shirt study', sniff tests showed that women prefer the odour of male perspiration when the man's tissue type is different to their own.[75] In real life, people have been shown to choose partners least likely to be related to them, based on the pheromones determined by their tissue type. The bad news is that these primitive pheromone messages are distorted by the use of the oral contraceptive pill and other chemical inputs.

I have heard one perfume scientist argue that women choose a perfume that 'enhances' their 'natural' smell. Surely an advocate for the fragrance industry! I think that he is wrong. To start with, the idea that modern artificial fragrances have any similarity to nature seems fanciful at best. And secondly, it would make more sense that a woman should choose a fragrance that *she* liked … the opposite of her own, thus giving out the wrong signal entirely.

It may be far-fetched, but could one factor in the high rates of marriage breakdown be the use of air fresheners in our cars and homes, and fragrances on our bodies?

COMMON ODOURS

'Wouldn't I know if it was making me sick, doctor?' Many patients know that the smell of cigarettes, cleaning agents, and perfumes will trigger a headache or a feeling of dysphoria. But most do not perceive these odours as noxious and are not made ill by them. Why is it that some people are?

Let us look at a common environmental poison.

Air freshener

I am sitting in with a young doctor on a teaching session. We hear a sound, like a gun being fired with a silencer on it. When I ask about it, I learn that it's the automatic room freshener, which apparently goes off every 15 minutes or so.

Having located the offending article and turned it off, I mentally note that I want to check exactly what substances it has been discharging into the confines of the room. I suspect that there will be 'fragrance', but what else?

When you learn about the 'what elses', it seems as if the human race has gone insane. Only the most optimistic among us could describe this chemical smog as 'freshening' anything. Chapter 3 looked at some poisons that are added to our foods, but even if we avoid eating them, we still have to breathe them in. When my Nanna (perfume notwithstanding) had a bad smell in the house, she opened a window. In a doctor's office, you might expect bad smells occasionally, and surely opening a window would be the best answer. Instead, this air 'freshener' has been discharging a cocktail of petrochemicals, whether they were needed or not, every 15 minutes.

I set out to do some research, and found that these are typical ingredients in air freshener.

- **Volatile organic compounds (VOCs):** Most of the chemicals discussed below under the heading 'Fragrance' are classified as volatile organic compounds. One of the more notorious VOCs in air freshener is formaldehyde.
- **Receptor blockers:** These compounds block the scent receptors in our noses and prevent us from detecting

certain noxious odours. (No kidding!)

- **Oxidants:** Yes, these are the very things we are trying to fight when we take antioxidants. You probably know the list of diseases with which they've been linked: arthritis, cancer, Parkinson's disease, and Alzheimer's, for starters. Examples of these oxidants include ozone, chlorate, chlorine, and hydrogen peroxide.

- **Sanitisers:** Air sanitisers, such as triethylene glycol, aim to inactivate airborne bacteria. A toxicity data sheet on triethylene glycol says: 'The substance is toxic to kidneys and the nervous system. Carcinogenic effects — *data not available*, Mutagenic effects — *data not available*, Teratogenic effects [causing malformations in a foetus] — *data not available*, Developmental effects — *data not available*.'[76] This stuff may be periodically sprayed on a pregnant patient in the doctor's surgery, or an expectant mother in her own home, and the possible effect of one of its ingredients on her unborn child is dismissed as 'data not available'?

- **'Maskers':** The term 'masker' can be applied to any substance that covers up a smell that industry has decided is too unpleasant for our delicate noses. The most commonly used masker is fragrance (discussed in detail shortly). These chemicals all add their toxins to this brew.

I will spare you an exhaustive list of the effects of these poisons on the brain, the nervous system, or a developing foetus. It is enough to note that headaches are among the side effects, and that cancer-causing chemicals are part of the deal. For what it is worth, a web search for formaldehyde and headache gave 99,000 hits; formaldehyde and migraine yielded 202,000 hits; formaldehyde and cluster headache, 7800; formaldehyde and tension headache, a mere 6500.

Global retail sales of air-care products, which include so-called air fresheners, were valued at more than $6 billion in 2006. That year, the US air-freshener market — comprising home air fresheners, car air fresheners, and potpourri — was worth $979.1 million, a 5.7 per cent increase on 2005 figures. (The largest segment, home air fresheners, made up around 91 per cent of the sales.)[77] The global sale of air fresheners has been forecast to reach $8.3 billion by 2015.[78]

We have just looked at the categories of chemicals involved. But let us look more closely at some of these ingredients, and some expert findings. We find formaldehyde, aerosol propellant, petroleum distillates, and p-dichlorobenzene. Then there are terpenes (a type of hydrocarbon) such as limonene, aldehydes, ketones, esters, alcohols, and synthetic fragrances. There is benzene, a classified human carcinogen. But the list does not end there. It includes styrene, phthalates, toluene, phosphates, chlorine bleach, and ammonia.[79]

A study of air fresheners by the US Natural Resources Defense Council found chemicals known to affect asthmatics, and known potential teratogens. The researchers recommended more rigorous supervision of the manufacturers. It seems that the law regards these chemicals as safe, and the public trusts the law. The US Food and Drug Administration's lists of foods that are generally regarded as safe are easily available, but things that we inhale as pollutants are not so easy to identify. You have to search chemical by chemical.

In 2009, Stanley M. Caress of the University of West Georgia and Anne C. Steinemann of the University of Washington looked at two epidemiological studies of health effects from exposure to air fresheners.[80] They found that nearly 20 per cent of all people and 34 per cent of asthmatics attributed headaches, breathing difficulties, or other symptoms to such exposure.

Fragrance

Walking through the perfume section of a department store is something of a nightmare for me. I could not have expressed it better than the author, Margaret Atwood, has in *Cat's Eye*:

> I revolve through revolving doors into [the store] ... The air is saturated with the stink of perfumes at war ... I stop only long enough to allow myself to be sprayed by a girl giving away free squirts of some venomous new perfume ... The stuff smells like grape Kool-Aid. I can't imagine it seducing anything but a fruit fly ... 'You like this?' I say to the girl ... 'It's been very popular,' she says evasively.

Perfume has been used since ancient times. The production of perfume was thought to have begun in that cradle of civilisation, Iran (or Persia, as it was known). Persian poet Omar Khayyám reminds us that Jamshid got hold of musk, ambergris, myrrh, camphor, saffron, and other sweet-smelling plants.[81]

We have references in the Bible to frankincense and myrrh,

which were rare and costly, but what of today's perfumes or fragrances? If you have ever suffered a headache induced by fragrance, you will know that it is almost impossible to avoid the smell. It emerges from your fellow passengers on the bus, in the interior of taxis, in luxury coaches, in conference washrooms, and from your colleagues and friends. Now even the boys are not safe: real men need perfume too, it seems. If we don't spray it on ourselves, we fill up the air we breathe with it. One specialist eye surgeon I know has asked his patients not to wear perfume when they come to see him. Perhaps he feels that operating on someone's eyes is risky enough, without a Picasso-like distortion in his own visual field.

So far I have not made this request of my patients because scent has become part of my diagnostic procedure. People often say that they don't wear perfume, because they don't include their deodorant or other cosmetics. My sensitivity to smell is a much better test.

Part of my teaching work has me travelling around the country and staying in hotels or motels. I have learned to request 'no air fresheners' as the result of one memorable occasion. I was exhausted after travelling all day. The motel reeked of cheap scent, and I knew I would spend the night inhaling petrochemicals. When I learnt that the advertised 'fresh coffee delivered to your room in the morning' was in fact instant coffee presented in a percolator pot, it was the last straw. I asked, 'Do you have any rooms that *don't* smell like a brothel?'

While rudeness can't ever be excused, I think my frustration can. If you're going to give me a headache, at least give me a decent caffeine fix to deal with it the next morning!

Many people experience headaches as a result of perfume. We know that up to a quarter of all women get migraines. What can you do when you've spent a week's salary to treat yourself to the opera and the person next to you is drenched in petrochemicals that will make you sick? Or you offer a friend a lift for a long journey and you get the headache aura the moment he steps into the car? One friend received correspondence from someone she knew to be a severe migraineur, and the pages were dense with the aroma of perfume. Even reading the correspondence gave my friend a headache, but the author was clearly unaware.

Let's return now to Catherine, from Chapter 1, and her migraine.

Catherine's story

Catherine, you remember, was a professional musician who suffered from recurrent migraines. She had found that milk and chocolate were triggers, and by giving them up, she had got rid of her headaches. I saw her only once in the following year, for a travel vaccine, and her headaches had not returned.

A few weeks later, I was surprised when my receptionist buzzed me to say that Catherine was on the phone, in agony with a headache. I made a home visit, and on entering her bedroom, I was stunned. The dressing table was covered from end to end with bottles of expensive perfume, bought duty-free when she toured. After getting over my shock, I said, 'Catherine, am I right in thinking that we have never had the perfume discussion?'

On the back of a stressful tour, a menstrual period, some unavoidable dairy exposure, and new bottles of duty-free perfume, the headaches were back as if they had never left. She was persuaded to add 'perfume' to 'milk and chocolate' on her list of addictive substances to avoid.

Catherine is not alone in failing to identify odours as a trigger of her headaches. Although some people make the link to perfume, petrol, and paints, and others volunteer that cigarette smoke makes them ill, many need to have their attention drawn to any possible connection. For those who wonder why they always get sick in smoky clubs and bars, the causes may include cigarette smoke, alcohol, and strobe lighting. But there are other possibilities: the perfume of their fellow merrymakers, carpets that exude flame-retardants, air fresheners in the bathrooms, and spray-on cleaning agents. We need to consider the role that all of these might play. When my Nanna wore perfume, she usually smelled of lavender (sometimes it was roses or violets, but mostly it was lavender). Although I found that it made me feel sick on car trips or when I had eaten chocolate, the rest of the time I thought she smelled nice.

I can imagine that even if you made a connection between your headaches and your perfume, you might endure it for the sake of smelling like flowers. But Mary's story highlights a puzzle: to my nostrils, most of the expensive modern 'fragrances' are anything but 'fragrant'. The word suggests something delicate drifting through the air, not a stench of vomit. Ironically, one expensive perfume has a name that's close to 'poison'.

So what are these 'poisons'? We have already looked at the toxic effect of the chemicals in air fresheners. The list overlaps with those found in fragrance. And do not assume that they will be listed on the bottle; manufacturers take it for granted that the word 'fragrance' will suffice. Space aside, who would want lists like the following on their product?

The National Academy of Science in the United States has estimated that about 95 per cent of a fragrance is made up of petrochemicals (or VOCs), including benzyl acetate, ethyl acetate, and benzaldehyde.[82] We can add the following groups to that list.

- **Persistent organic pollutants (POPs):** These chemicals, such as benzyl acetate and benzaldehyde, are often used in agriculture to control pests and diseases. Some are banned, but they have such long half-lives that they continue to pollute the food chain and the environment long after the bans come into effect. The US Environment Protection Agency found that synthetic musk compounds from perfume and cosmetics were pervasive; they occur in the sediment of the Great Lakes, and even in the milk of breastfeeding mothers.[83]

- **Phthalates:** These are usually labelled as such. In industry, they are used as plasticisers, and in many cosmetics, they are used to make fragrance 'last longer'. They have a known pro-oestrogenic and anti-androgenic effect, and have been linked to sperm damage. They are also suspected carcinogens.

- **Polycyclic aromatic hydrocarbons (PAHs):** These are produced by the heating of coal, oil, gas, and wood. Mineral oil, which appears in commercial creams, lotions, and even baby cream, is a byproduct of the distillation of crude oil into gasoline.

- **Volatile organic compounds (VOCs):** Already mentioned, VOCs are organic solvents that out-gas easily into the surrounding air. Most of the following ingredients are classified as VOCs, and they are the main components of all fragrances. Formaldehyde and limonene are examples of VOCs that have been linked to irritation and headache. Formaldehyde is a suspected carcinogen.

Some specific examples of these chemicals found in fragrance include the following.

- **Acetone:** Found in cologne, detergent, and nail-polish remover. Primary toxic medical effects include nausea, dizziness, slurred speech, and central nervous system depression. It is classified as a VOC.
- **Benzaldehyde:** Found in products such as perfume, cologne, hairspray, laundry bleach, deodorants, detergent, Vaseline, shaving cream, shampoo, bar soap, and dishwasher detergent. Toxic effects include nausea and abdominal pain, central nervous system depression, possible kidney damage, and narcotic effects. (Perhaps my patients really *do* get addicted to this stuff!)
- **Benzyl acetate:** Found in cosmetics, this is a known respiratory irritant. It is linked to pancreatic cancer — which is showing a worrying rise in the Western world, for no known reason.
- **Benzyl alcohol:** Found in products such as perfume, deodorant, Vaseline, shampoo, nail-polish remover,

and air freshener. Toxic effects include headaches,
nausea, vomiting, dizziness, a drop in blood pressure,
and central nervous system depression.

- **Camphor:** Found in products such as perfume, shaving
  cream, fabric softener, dishwasher detergent, nail
  polish, and air freshener. It can cause dizziness, nausea,
  confusion, and convulsions. Has been fatal to babies
  wrapped in bedding exposed to it.

- **Ethanol:** Found in products such as perfume, hairspray,
  shampoo, fabric softener, dishwashing liquid, and
  detergent. Effects include agitation and drowsiness,
  dizziness and confusion; it also has effects on the
  central nervous system, including headaches. If
  alcohol gives you a headache, don't be surprised if
  the ethanol in fragrance does too. It's the same stuff.
  Remember that it's also a solvent and a fuel substitute
  that you are spraying around.

- **Ethyl acetate:** Found in products such as aftershave,
  cologne, perfume, shampoo, nail polish, nail-polish
  remover, fabric softener, and dishwashing liquid. It has
  a narcotic effect, producing headaches and stupor, as
  well as causing anaemia and blood disorders, and liver
  and kidney damage.

- **Linalool:** This ubiquitous chemical is found in
  products such as perfume, cologne, bar soap,
  shampoo, hand lotion, nail-polish remover, hairspray,
  laundry detergent, dishwashing liquid, Vaseline, air
  fresheners, bleach powder, fabric softener, shaving
  cream, aftershave, and solid deodorant. Toxic effects
  are seen in the central nervous system and are

classified as narcotic. It can cause headaches and has an 'addictive' effect.

- **Methylene chloride:** This one is found in products such as shampoo, cologne, and paint and varnish remover. According to my references, it was 'banned by the US Food and Drug Administration in 1988', but '*no enforcement [was] possible due to trade secret laws protecting chemical fragrance industry*' (my italics).[84] It appears on the hazardous waste lists published by the US Environmental Protection Agency and in two pieces of US legislation, the *Resource Conservation and Recovery Act* and the *Comprehensive Environmental Response, Compensation, and Liability Act*. It is listed as a carcinogen; other toxic effects include headache, fatigue, irritability, and central nervous system disorders.

- **G-terpinene:** Found in products such as cologne, perfume, soap, shaving cream, deodorant, and air freshener. It can cause asthma and disorders of the central nervous system.

- **A-terpineol:** Found in products such as perfume, cologne, laundry detergent, bleach powder, laundry bleach, fabric softener, air freshener, Vaseline, cologne, soap, hairspray, aftershave, and roll-on deodorant. It is said to be highly irritating to mucous membranes and can cause excitation, ataxia, hypothermia, depression of the central nervous system and the respiratory system, and headache.[85]

So there seem to be a lot of these chemicals around?
My response is to quote the bestselling book *Slow Death by Rubber Duck*: 'By the time the average woman grabs her morning coffee, she has applied 126 different chemicals in 12 different products to her face, body and hair.'[86]

And what are all these chemicals doing to me?
Environmental chemicals, both the ones in your food and the ones you inhale, might help explain some of your other health problems, besides headaches. Chapter 1 looked at many health problems known to be associated with headaches. Several of those have a clear link to what you might be breathing in.

What about to others?
In a shocking postscript to this discussion, in late 2013, as I was preparing the final drafts for this book, I read over my morning coffee a headline: 'With a Whiff of Eau de Baby'.[87] As I continued on in horror, I learnt that there is a 'booming baby perfume market'. Designed to 'enhance' a baby's natural odour, the product is intended to disguise the smells of sour milk, dirty nappies, and vomit. Worth exposing your baby to hormone-disrupting chemicals and carcinogens, priming its NMDA receptors, I wonder?

What can be done?
I don't know how we solve this. Some patients, such as Mary and Catherine, will try anything. Others are so attached to their perfume that nothing will persuade them. Or they will stop wearing the perfume, but still get sick from the lingering

fragrance on their clothes. There seems to be no solution for the VOCs and other compounds that permeate the air we breathe. As far as I can see, two forms of action are possible: activism and education.

Activism

Products like air fresheners and fragrances are a big industry in themselves, and they form part of an even bigger industry: the petrochemical industry. When you use perfume, you are spraying a petroleum product on yourself. Politicians will not tackle the big end of town unless forced to do so by public opinion. But it seems that only a minority of the public think there is a problem; the majority don't care. Only activism will bring about change.

Despite the cries of 'perfume police', sufferers of headaches, multiple chemical sensitivity, and chronic fatigue syndrome are slowly making airborne chemicals a health and safety issue. The battle began in the late 1990s and is proving to be as bitter as that against public smoking. In 2004, the Canadian city of Halifax, in Nova Scotia, instituted a policy to discourage the wearing of fragrance in public buildings. By 2010, an impressive list of public institutions were promoting fragrance-free environments.[88] Since 2007, students at California State University have been pushing for a fragrance-free campus. Similar action has been taken at Cecil College in Maryland and Portland State University.[89]

In Chapter 5, we saw that a study had shown an alarming doubling of the rate of stroke in young women since 1995. It is impossible to nail a single cause for this, but if we could show a link to the increased usage of perfumes and 'air fresheners', surely something would have to be done. Years ago, you wore perfume on a special date; now people are inhaling it for breakfast.

Education

I try to educate my patients and hope that they will give me a hearing. A website called ScentSense is also very helpful.[90]

But ignorance about airborne chemicals is widespread. Even those who might be expected to understand the issue seem blind to the problem. In a recent radio interview, Professor Andrew Charles, Director of Headache Research and Treatment at the University of California in Los Angeles, outlined a systematic approach to headache management, covering neurology, anatomy, biochemistry, therapeutics, and lifestyle. He did not mention the avoidance of chemicals. My frustration at this was echoed by one online commenter, 'JB', who wrote: 'I find it interesting that hypersensitivity to smells is rarely mentioned ... This is particularly true of perfume.'[91]

I become emotional when I consider the headache clinics (and, indeed, cancer clinics) that fail to recognise, let alone address, the problems of environmental chemicals. I am distressed by the millions of research dollars that are spent trying to find the magic cure to problems that might have simple causes in everyday chemicals. It is perverse to seek a 'cure' while questions of causation stare us in the face. Medical education produces doctors who fail to see that headaches, autism, and cancer may all flourish in the chemical soup that we live in.

When individuals, or the doctors who treat those suffering from chronic fatigue syndrome or chronic headaches, do not make the connection between their condition and indoor air quality and fragrance, how can we expect the politicians to do so?

Natural perfumes

Sometimes people ask about essential oils and 'natural' perfumes. We need to understand that when nature creates a perfume, it is a compound of aromatics, aldehydes (a form of organic compound), and terpenes. Nature does this for a reason: the plant is trying to send a message through its pheromone system. The message may be 'come on', or 'stay away', or something else again. A recent *New Scientist* headline puts this bluntly: 'Sweet Scent Doubles as Repellent for Flower Eaters'.[92] Chemically sensitive people may react to something that is purely attractive to someone else. My mother loved the smell of gardenias, but she developed both hay fever and migraine if they were brought into the house. Some patients have commented that heavily perfumed flowers, such as hibiscus, jasmine, or lilac, can provoke such a reaction in them, too. Here there can be no specific advice. For ourselves, we may need to consider fresh flowers when we are looking at triggers for headaches. For others, we should be sensitive to the possibility that not everyone has a pleasant response to flower fragrances.

We have just seen that some human-made chemicals have pro-oestrogenic and anti-androgenic effects. Patients with hormonally driven cancers, such as ovarian, breast, and prostate cancer, should stay away from cosmetics containing these chemicals. Infertile couples should too. *The New England Journal of Medicine* warns against the use of lavender and tea-tree oils for the same reason.[93] They have been linked to gynecomastia (tender breast swelling) in young boys, indicating that their chemical activities include significant endocrine disruption. While this does not specifically link to headaches in these boys, it highlights just how powerful odours can be, even if they are entirely natural.

I think of a patient who felt oppressed and headachy whenever she walked into a rainforest. Rainforests are a rich mix of smells, ranging from pollens through to moulds and terpenes. Moulds in particular have a strong smell, often quite unpleasant. My patient's headaches could easily be understood in these terms. It is safe to say that nature's plant smells, although they contain various levels of compounds from the chemical classes above, are less likely to cause headaches than synthetic products. But every person will react differently.[94] My patient chose to avoid walking in forests. I think this is a pity, and may be missing the point. If the gun wasn't loaded, and if there were locks on the triggers, could she expect a different experience?

Cigarette smoke

The larger part of this chapter has focused on chemically manufactured odours. And we have discussed natural odours, such as those from flowers, and from moulds or rainforests. But it would be a major omission not to conclude with one of the most toxic odours of all: cigarette smoke. While tobacco is natural, exposure to the carcinogens and other chemicals in burnt tobacco cannot be thought of as 'natural'.

Many patients report tobacco smoke, either from their own smoking or secondhand smoke, as a precipitant of their headaches. Indeed, third-hand smoke — an encounter with clothes worn by a smoker, or a hotel room previously used by a smoker — has been implicated. The smoke may be that of cigarettes, cigars, or pipes. While marijuana has sometimes been touted as a treatment for migraine, others report that it can trigger their headaches. Headaches particularly associated with smoking include migraine and cluster.

Like fragrance, this is a matter of individual preference. People must like some of these odours, or they would not go out of their way to surround themselves with them. And to end on a curiously perverse note, I find myself attracted to the smell of many cigars, though it's been decades since I have tried a puff of one!

CHAPTER 8
Taking Control: nutritional supplements and healthy living

'No problem is too small or too trivial if we can really do something about it.'
RICHARD FEYNMAN

Let's return to the analogy that compares headaches to a loaded gun. If you've got the headaches, we can infer the existence of the gun, which is probably genetic. You can't alter your headache gun, but you choose whether you load it with bullets, whether you pull the trigger, or, indeed, whether you put a safety catch on the trigger.

But first, a word of warning. 'Natural' medications such as vitamins, minerals, and herbs are generally fairly safe, but they should only be used after a proper medical assessment has ruled out such conditions as brain tumour and stroke. In all cases, ongoing supervision by qualified professionals is recommended.

GETTING STARTED

- First, visit your doctor for a clear diagnosis. If you've never seen a neurologist, ask for a referral.
- Ask your doctor for relevant blood tests. Consider paying for tests for iron studies, MTHFR genotyping, and vitamin D, homocysteine, vitamin B12, and folate levels. Also consider getting IgG food sensitivity tests. Check your serum copper level: high levels are associated with headaches in some people.
- Pay attention to any gut problems. Full treatment of this topic is beyond the scope of this book, but if you have 'funny guts' or digestive problems, they need to be sorted out. Maybe it is one of the food intolerances we have discussed, or maybe it something to do with abnormal bugs in your gut. (See more on this in Chapters 11 and 13.)
- Seek help from your doctor or naturopath to undertake an elimination diet. (See more on this in Chapter 6.)
- Visit your dentist and ask whether you need treatment for bruxism, malocclusion, or problems in the temporo-mandibular joint (TMJ).

My suggestion is that you start simply. Choose a diet, don't wear perfume, and take a magnesium supplement.

The following are some simple checklists to provide some guidance on other things you may wish to do. With the exception of the information regarding your chosen diet, don't feel obliged to follow all the advice at once. It can be both confusing and restrictive.

Avoid bullets and triggers

Consider whether any of the following might play a role in your headaches, and work out how you can change your routine to avoid them:

- alcohol and cigarettes (in any amount)
- excess salt
- food additives and preservatives
- foods that you are sensitive to
- household chemicals, paints, and sprays
- lighting (fluorescent lights, strobe lighting, compact fluorescent tubes, and household lighting at the blue-white end of the light spectrum; aim for 'warm white' and yellow tones)
- overuse of medication
- perfume or cosmetics
- recreational drugs.

Gut health

Hippocrates famously said that all diseases begin in the gut, and we saw in Chapter 1 that irritable bowel syndrome has links to migraine. The neurotransmitters discussed throughout this book have many receptors in the gut.

Chronic bowel problems may cause your headaches, or be a clue as to the cause. You may need medical help or advice from a naturopath.

Herbs

More detail on these to follow shortly, but the key ones to mention are feverfew, which is commonly used for migraine (preparations are found widely in health food shops), and ginger, which is especially useful for nausea.

Psychological health

If there are issues in your relationships, try to identify and deal with them. Counsellors, psychologists, and psychotherapists are all used to dealing with people with chronic stress problems.

Do a cost–benefit analysis, preferably with such a therapist. Is your health really the price you are willing to pay to stay in a destructive relationship or a toxic work environment?

Some problems, such as grief and loss, don't have 'answers', but talk therapy in its various guises has demonstrable health benefits.

Physical therapies

In every health problem where studies have been done, exercise has been shown to be of benefit. Make it part of your normal routine. However, do not try to exercise while you have a serious headache.

Visit a chiropractor or physiotherapist to see if you have postural problems that may be playing a role in your headaches and need attention.

Relaxation techniques

Perhaps the source of your stress is unavoidable, such as ageing and dependent relatives, chronic illness in yourself or loved ones, natural disasters, and so on. However, your neural responses to those stresses can be modified by various approaches.

Consider hypnosis, meditation, yoga, tai chi, remedial massage, listening to or playing music, or prayer. Creative or artistic activities can have a similar effect; make time for them. Also consider learning about biofeedback techniques that help you to induce relaxing alpha waves.

Vitamins and minerals

These are discussed in more detail shortly, but here is a quick list of useful supplements.

- **B vitamins:** These are often found as multi-B preparations. Especially important are B2 (riboflavin; may require large doses), B6, B12, and B9 (folic acid).
- **Coenzyme Q10 (CoQ10):** Try taking 150-milligram capsules once daily for at least three months.
- **Essential fatty acids:** Both fish oil and evening primrose oil preparations are useful and widely available.
- **Magnesium:** This should preferably be an amino acid chelate, magnesium orotate, or magnesium citrate, but good effects have also been found with magnesium sulphate.
- **Tiger Balm ointment:** Applied topically, it is as effective as standard medication in treating tension headache.
- **Vitamin D:** Check blood levels first, and if deficient, take 1000 to 5000 international units (IU) daily.

THE ROLE OF NUTRITIONAL SUPPLEMENTS

Nature has all kinds of inbuilt safety mechanisms to protect us from the environmental challenges we might meet, and the tendency for headaches is no exception. In the gun analogy, nutritional supplements can act as a safety catch on the trigger, giving your body more resilience against the factors that set off your headaches.

A trigger may be something as fundamental as lack of sleep, or it may be a lack of vitamins, minerals, or essential fatty acids.

B vitamins

Chapter 2 discussed a trial by Lyn Griffiths and her team at Griffith University's Genomics Research Centre, which showed that people with certain variants of the MTHFR and MTRR genes found their headaches were helped by taking extra vitamin B12 and folic acid. Those with a double dose of this gene, you will remember, had the least benefit from the supplements. If you are one of these, you should try to overcome the 'roadblock' with 5-MTHF (the active form of folic acid, also known as levomefolic acid), and possibly folinic acid (an alternative form of folic acid, also known as leucovorin). These two may need a prescription, and may need to be supplied by a compounding pharmacist.

Other studies have indicated a role for high-dose vitamin B2 (riboflavin) in migraine prophylaxis and possibly treatment. In 2004, Sydney neurologist Doctor Alessandro Zagami successfully trialled subjects with 400 milligrams of riboflavin daily for six months.[95] The recommended daily intake for vitamin B2 is around 1.5 milligrams, so the vitamin was being used in pharmacological (drug-like) quantities. Without funding for long-term safety studies, this must remain a provisional recommendation.

The reason for the beneficial effect of these large doses of riboflavin was thought to be support for impaired mitochondrial function. Riboflavin has also been shown to inhibit the release of glutamate from nerve terminals in the brain of rats.[96] In view of the role of glutamate in the headache attack (Chapter 12), if the findings can be extrapolated to humans, the benefits are obvious.

Even at normal doses, riboflavin may work by another means and have another useful application. Vitamin B2 is a co-factor for the MTHFR gene. This means that if you have a less functional polymorphism of this gene, vitamin B2 will help it work better. A 2010 study showed that people with a double dose of the MTHFR C>T polymorphism and evidence of low vitamin B2 could lower their blood pressure by a significant degree when supplemented with just 1.6 milligrams of riboflavin daily.[97] This amount is often present in a healthy diet, but not always. As longstanding migraine is a marker for an increased risk of stroke and cardiovascular disease, the value of B2 supplementation is worth considering.

Essential fatty acids

These are the 'good oils', such as omega-3 and omega-6 fatty acids. In a primitive diet, the ratio between these two kinds of good oil was about even. Now our diets contain about 16 omega-6 fatty acids to one omega-3.[98] Even good oils can become 'bad' at this level of imbalance; it can lead to inflammation, which promotes the chemicals that can trigger headache and pain. We need more omega-3s in our diet. Fish oil, flaxseed oil, and walnuts are good sources.[99]

Herbs

We tend to think of herbs as natural medicines, and Mother Nature laced our foods with herbal medicines.[100] We cannot separate food and medicine. In our modern diet, much of nature's bounty is left out, and we have to resort to the medicine chest far more often than we ought.

Every culture of medical therapy has herbal remedies for headache. If your headaches are intractable, investigate Ayurvedic, Chinese, and Tibetan medicines. Recommendations for herbal medicines are beyond my expertise, but practitioners of these disciplines can be found readily in any city or large town.

Some studies of other modalities done according to Western techniques show impressive results. One such was on the use of Tiger Balm for tension headaches, carried out by Monash University in Melbourne.[101] The effects of fresh ginger, coriander, lavender, peppermint, chamomile, rosehip, valerian root, and feverfew have also all been studied. Some of these herbs can be drunk as teas, while others are used in dried form in sachets applied to the forehead. Peppermint, for example, either as a tea or in lolly form, is claimed to help nausea or stomach pain. Ginger contains 5-HT3 antagonists (see Chapter 9), gingerols, and shogaols, making it a useful anti-emetic (something that helps to alleviate vomiting and nausea). Capsaicin, the active ingredient in chilli and cayenne pepper, has been tried on a wide range of headaches with good reports. Feverfew is a herb with a long record of migraine relief. No doubt a herbalist could tell you about others.

Even so-called magic mushrooms have recently been studied for the treatment of depression. The thinking goes like this. Psychedelics are traditionally thought of as stimulating activity in the brain, but in fact they suppress excess activity in certain critical areas. Psilocybin (the naturally occurring psychedelic compound in some species of mushrooms) seems to do this by reducing blood flow to the hypothalamus. But there is also considerable anecdotal evidence that some sufferers of cluster headaches, and maybe migraineurs, can get benefit. Will the medical boffins countenance clinical trials that use 'illegal substances' for depression and cluster headache?

More information about herbs that can help to treat headaches is easy to find online; also see below.

Magnesium

Supplements containing magnesium have been beneficial across the spectrum of headache sufferers. A good balanced diet tends to have a reasonable amount of magnesium. Magnesium is important in different genetic variants, as we have seen.

Although a fully natural diet has only marginally more calcium than magnesium, we have seen that the Western diet often has eight times more calcium than magnesium. Modern agriculture creates an imbalance by using artificial fertilisers, and our dietary choices can make this worse. If you have the genes that are affected by such an imbalance, you are more likely to get headaches. A study published in *Cephalalgia* in 1996 showed the benefit of magnesium citrate in preventing migraine.[102] Among other actions, it made certain receptors less sensitive to glutamate. Magnesium was putting a lock on the trigger.

Even if we do not know our genotype, it's a good precautionary measure to make sure that our diets are rich in these safety catches. And we should always regard supplementing as something to be done with the appropriate professional guidance.

TREATMENTS FOR NAUSEA

As nausea and vomiting are unpleasant parts of many headaches, it is worth seeking out natural treatments. Ginger and peppermint have already been mentioned. Both the over-the-counter medication Emetrol and the chemical muscimol are claimed to have anti-emetic properties. Another purported anti-emetic is ajwain, a spice popular in India, Ethiopia, and Eritrea.[103]

Dosage

The suggestions that follow carry the same caveat of medical supervision as at the beginning of this chapter. As the Australian Therapeutic Goods Administration allows almost all of the following to be sold as over-the-counter preparations, we can assume that their use is regarded as safe. The exceptions to over-the-counter sale are the high-dose vitamin

B2, folinic acid, and folic acid in the form of 5-MTHF. These can be sold by registered naturopaths, or by compounding pharmacies with a doctor's prescription.

So what do you recommend I take?

In the scenario I outlined at the beginning of Chapter 2, this question would be a lot easier to answer. I would know your genetic vulnerabilities, and know where the emphasis should lie. Various supplements have been mentioned throughout this book, and many of them are backed by clinical trials — some of which meet at least the criteria required by mainstream medical investigation.

I start patients on magnesium, progressively adding the other supplements in the order listed.

Magnesium

I suggest taking 250 to 400 milligrams three times a day. The usual recommendation is to use an amino acid chelate, such as magnesium orotate or aspartate. The trials referenced by *Cephalalgia* in Chapter 2 used magnesium citrate. In Chapter 12, I also make a case for using magnesium sulphate. Magnesium oxide is much cheaper than magnesium sulphate, but is poorly absorbed by the body. However, any of these options could be tried.

Some studies have used magnesium sulphate given intravenously. Intravenous administration is carried out by medical practitioners, of course; self-administration, or administration by anyone other than a fully trained medical doctor, would be very dangerous.

Essential B vitamins

The basic requirements are for B6, B12, and folic acid. You need advice from a pharmacist or naturopath to make sure you get the doses right. The trial conducted at Griffith University used 2 milligrams of folic acid, 25 milligrams of B6, and 400 micrograms of B12. These supplements are easily available over the counter at pharmacies and good health-food stores.

If you have been tested for the MTHFR gene mutation and are homozygous for the mutated form, instead of the folic acid, you may benefit from the special form of folic acid discussed above: namely, 5-MTHF, at doses of 5 or more milligrams daily, and/or 500 micrograms of folinic acid daily. These will need prescription by a medical practitioner who is used to prescribing them. In Australia, trained naturopaths are licensed to sell low-dose versions of these supplements.

Extra B vitamins

Some people will benefit from extra vitamin B2 (riboflavin): between 200 and 400 milligrams daily. It must be noted that this is a pharmacological dose — that is, a massive dose never found in nature. This should be trialled for three months. High-dose riboflavin is available from some pharmacies and some health-food stores where there is a naturopath onsite to give advice. Medical supervision is advised.

Coenzyme Q10

I suggest taking 150 milligrams of CoQ10 daily for three months. If this seems to help, continue with it, as it is generally regarded as safe.[104]

Fish-oil capsules

I suggest taking three to six 1000-milligram capsules daily. Headaches are connected with inflammatory cytokines, and fish oil, which contains omega-3 fatty acids, is anti-inflammatory. A fish-based diet is even better.

Vitamin D

Vitamin D is a pain modulator considered relevant in migraine and chronic tension-type headaches. Get your vitamin D levels tested to make sure that you stay in a good range. Those who are shown to be deficient should take up to 5000 international units daily: the usual replacement dose is 1000 international units daily, and this will be adequate for many people, but some will need higher doses. The higher doses are safe so long as you get regular blood tests to ensure that they have not reached toxic levels.

Investigators presented the results of an observational study at the 50th annual meeting of the American Headache Society, which showed that 41.8 per cent of patients with chronic migraine were deficient in 25-hydroxy vitamin D. The study also showed that the longer individuals had chronic migraine, the more likely they were to be deficient in vitamin D.[105]

Penelope's story

As Penelope came through my door, I smelled the perfume. It would have been hard not to. Like many people, she would reapply it several times during the day if she felt that it was 'wearing off'.

Penelope was in her forties and had been diagnosed at a

headache clinic as having 'classic migraine', with hormonal exacerbation. She was on a range of medications, and when her period was due, she was in the habit of setting an alarm for 4 a.m. to take some of these. Penelope worked as a nurse, but had not done shift work in years. She had a responsible position as a ward manager and hated to ring in sick. Her husband, who worked for an airline, could bring home lots of duty-free fancy perfumes.

I started Penelope on magnesium, and we had the diet discussion. A non-smoker and a non-drinker, she said that chocolate was her only vice, although she only ate a small amount each night. When I added that of course there could be no perfume worn during the trial period, I realised that there *was* another 'vice'. She could just about imagine going without chocolate for a while, but she could *not* imagine life without perfume.

When I saw her next, the smell of fragrance was still there. She denied using it since the last visit, so I suggested that she might have to wash items of clothing that might be holding the fumes. At the first consultation, Penelope had commented that when she experienced stress at work, she would feel her jaw tighten and her neck muscles stiffen. If a period was due, the headaches would often break through no matter how much medication she took. She would wake with an aching jaw, and her husband had told her that he could hear her grinding her teeth in the night. A visit to the dentist had resulted in a splint for her bruxism. She felt that this was helping the headaches 'somewhat'.

As the headaches slowly lessened, the next step was to try to reduce her medication. But it soon became clear that this was leading to rebound headaches. Changing the environment is one thing; dealing with the iatrogenic (doctor-induced) effect is another. Both doctor and patient need to go slowly. Eventually, we got there.

My last consultation with Penelope was poignant: not realising my own sensitivity to perfumes, she asked whether I wanted a suitcase full of Chanel No. 5 and similar perfumes (worth thousands of dollars, I gather). I graciously declined. By then she was entirely headache-free, sleeping with her dental brace every night and not on any medication. As she left the room, she also told me triumphantly that she was back eating chocolate as before, with no problems!

Tension headaches? Migraine? Hormonal? You can decide.

After a couple of months of implementing the changes outlined in this chapter, many people report themselves 'cured' or significantly better. Several feel confident to experiment with various other interventions. In some cases, the headaches have improved, but they still need help in reducing the medications.

If there has been little change, I suggest that you and your doctor get a second opinion from another doctor with a lot of experience in practising this kind of medicine. (A contact list of Australian doctors is in Appendix 2, along with some overseas links.) You may need a review from a specialist neurologist. Two heads are usually better than one.

One of my patients adhered to all that we have just discussed. There was no progress at all. I sent him to a colleague who was very experienced in food intolerances, thinking that she might be able to nail it. She later said, 'I just didn't like the look of him.' He looked pale and pasty. I had put that appearance down to hours spent in front of a computer, the 'nerdy' lifestyle. She diagnosed a clostridial bowel infection. After she had treated him for this infection, the headaches went.

CHAPTER 9
Medication: from common drugs to complex prescriptions

'Oh well done! I commend your pains,
And every one shall share i' th' gains.'
HECATE, A WITCH IN 'MACBETH'

Let us begin by looking at what your GP needs to take into account when deciding which drugs to prescribe for your headaches. We'll concentrate primarily on migraine, but will not confine ourselves to this headache. I have divided the medications into 'acute' phase medications and 'preventive' or interim treatments. I also look at some of the disadvantages of these drugs.

It has to be stressed that I am not recommending any of these treatments. Many of the medications require a prescription from your doctor anyway. Nor should you use the following information to change or combine your prescribed medications; it is solely for the purpose of knowing more about what you have been or may be prescribed. Furthermore, even products such as aspirin and paracetamol, which can be bought over the counter, should only be taken after a doctor has assessed you. In all cases, ongoing supervision by qualified medical professionals is recommended.

COMMON HEADACHE DRUGS

A familiarity with the names of common headache drugs will help you to understand how they work.

Firstly, you will notice that some drugs are described as 'antagonists' and others as 'agonists': for instance, there are both serotonin agonists and serotonin antagonists.

- Antagonists try to *block* a substance, such as serotonin. Or they may block the receptor for that substance, producing a similar outcome. Some of the key ingredients in medications listed below, such as methysergide and cyproheptadine, act as serotonin antagonists, and are used to *prevent* migraine.
- Agonists try to *mimic* the substance in question, or to activate it. Triptans, for example, are employed as serotonin receptor agonists (at the time of a headache).

This is confusing, and the reason for the confusion is that the actions of neurotransmitters such as serotonin and its various receptors are complex and diverse. Moreover, different serotonin receptors create different effects. And preventing a headache is not the same as treating it once it has happened.

Drugs for treating an acute attack

Drugs have a role to play in treating the various symptoms of headache.

Simple analgesics

The first-line treatment for all headaches is usually a simple analgesic, such as paracetamol or aspirin. Some people find that these are effective, and their main concern is whether they are taking too many. Aspirin can have a good effect in some cases because it reduces platelet stickiness and, as we saw in the discussion of the vascular theory in Chapter 5, some migraines represent mini-strokes.[106]

However, many people say of these analgesics, 'They just don't touch me, doctor.'

Anti-inflammatories

Next in line are the drugs known as non-steroidal anti-inflammatory drugs, or NSAIDs. Typical medications in this group include Naprosyn, Brufen, and Nurofen. Some people, including migraineurs, find them very effective. NSAIDs are the first-line treatment for paroxysmal hemicrania (see Chapter 10). Other people, even though they find the medications effective in relieving pain, have trouble tolerating them because of complications such as aspirin-sensitive asthma, gastric irritation, or bleeding.

NSAIDs are available over the counter and even in supermarkets, despite the gravity of the side effects. I have never understood how the Australian Therapeutic Goods Administration and similar international bodies came to this decision, and to this day I disagree with it on safety grounds. These drugs often play a role in headaches *caused* by medication overuse.

Sedatives

If the patient is able to sleep, sedative medications may be helpful. In Australia, the drug Mersyndol is often prescribed, and in the United Kingdom, a similar product called Migraleve can be used. These drugs combine codeine and paracetamol to provide analgesia, with an antihistamine as a sedative. In Mersyndol, the antihistamine is doxylamine succinate; in Migraleve, it is buclizine.

These old-style antihistamines are well known for sedation. However, histamine itself is a neurotransmitter linked to headaches (see Chapters 6, 10, and 12). The antihistamines may relieve pain not only through their sedative effect but also directly, because they block the release of histamine.

These combination medications have been used for both migraine and tension headaches. Many patients tolerate them well because of the absence of aspirin or NSAIDs.

Ergot derivatives

The next group of medications includes ergotamine tartrate and dihydroergotamine (see Chapters 1 and 12). These drugs have long been in use for migraine and cluster headaches. As we have already seen, they are derived from ergot alkaloids.

Historically, ergot alkaloids in a fungus known to grow on rye have been identified as a cause of poisoning. The poison causes constriction of blood vessels, and so it has been regarded as a logical solution for the dilated, throbbing vessels of the scalp and brain. As well as constricting cranial blood vessels, ergots may also have an effect on the pain pathways. It is thought that ergotamine medication may activate receptors in the periaqueductal grey matter, or PAG (see Chapter 11). Like the triptans discussed shortly, ergot derivatives probably act as selective serotonin agonists.

Some medications combine ergot with caffeine and either an antihistamine or an anti-emetic (see below). Over time, ergot preparations have included tablets, suppositories, inhalers, and nasal sprays. Until the introduction of the triptans, ergot derivatives were the mainstay of treatment for severe migraine. I do not prescribe this class of drugs, partly because of the ease with which they lead to dependence or addiction. The addiction does not provide any sort of high that would appeal to the recreational drug user, but dependence can develop rapidly. Patients who use ergot regularly find that, although the drug relieves their headache, they need more of it and more often. Although some neurologists give formulas for the amount or frequency needed to run the risk of dependence, I think that this is too simplistic. Genetic variables already mentioned render such generalisations of limited value. Some define ergot dependence as when the drug is being used on more than ten days in a month. Many patients who take ergot, when I see them, are using it daily. Furthermore, I have found that ergot withdrawal is one of the most common causes of rebound or 'medication overuse' headaches, and one of the hardest to treat.

A recent edition of the *British National Formulary*, a drug information bible for doctors in the United Kingdom, states:

'Ergot alkaloids are rarely required now; oral and rectal preparations are associated with many side-effects, and they should be avoided in cerebrovascular or cardiac disease.'[107] I could not agree more. Nonetheless, ergot derivatives are still seen as one of the mainstays of migraine management in many places.

Side effects of ergot alkaloids include nausea, vomiting, diarrhoea, and, as mentioned, rebound headaches. Some people react with whitening and numbness of the fingertips as small blood vessels constrict, similar to the condition known as Raynaud's phenomenon. Ergot derivatives should not be given to patients with basilar or hemiplegic migraine, ischaemic heart disease, significant hypertension, or peripheral vascular diseases.

As discussed in Chapter 2, many migraine sufferers carry mutations of the MTHFR gene and its associated risks of vascular spasm and stroke. The use of ergot in such patients is worrying, and encourages us to look for safer treatments. Currently, neither they nor their doctors are likely to be aware of their MTHFR status.

Ergot with caffeine

Some ergot preparations contain caffeine, which aids in the constriction of arteries. Caffeine can also can stimulate gastric activity, which is seen as beneficial because it promotes the absorption of other medications.

Some patients say that drinking coffee relieves their headaches; others say that caffeine *gives* them a headache. Neither response surprises me. Caffeine binds to the adenosine receptor in the brain. Current research is focusing on the role of adenosine receptors, not only in migraine, but also in sleep disturbance and other brain disorders. The receptors come in various polymorphisms, and because they are activated by alcohol, there are genetic factors that might alter your sensitivity to alcohol. We will discuss these receptors more in Chapter 13, but let us look at caffeine more closely now.

Chapter 3 discussed the alkaloid effects of coffee. Other recent research has looked at this from a different point of view, studying the use of caffeine and aspirin in 'migraine-prone' rats. Originally I was riveted by the image of a rat nursing a migraine, but what I found even more interesting was the study's insight into alcohol sensitivity. Many migraineurs report that even one drink will give them a headache. This study describes how rats that are prone to migraine developed signs of headache when given even very small amounts of alcohol. It turned out that the rats appeared to be responding to acetate — one of the breakdown products of alcohol. Acetate activates the adenosine receptors. Both caffeine and aspirin block the effects of acetate, and this would explain why patients often stumble on the caffeine treatment for themselves.[108]

Anti-emetics

Nausea and vomiting often accompany headaches and may warrant treatment in their own right. Two widely used drugs are chlorpromazine (the key ingredient in brands such as Largactil) and prochlorperazine (the key ingredient in brands such as Stemetil), and they belong to a family known as phenothiazines. They act as dopamine antagonists, reducing both pain and nausea in migraine. Side effects are mild and include constipation, dizziness, and a dry mouth. But they can include truly alarming side effects in the extrapyramidal system, which include involuntary movements, such as those often associated with cerebral palsy. Or there may be an inability to initiate movement. Sometimes the person appears to be having a fit — frightening to both the victim and the onlookers.

Maxalon (metoclopramide) and Motilium (domperidome) are related medications used to reduce nausea and to increase the absorption of further medications from the stomach. They have similar side effects.

Cyclizine is a medication from the antihistamine family, and is used in combination with ergot medications, or may be used on its own for motion sickness, vertigo, and labyrinthine (ear canal) disorders. For more on nausea and vomiting, see Chapter 13.

Here is a more complete list of anti-emetics.

- Dopamine antagonists, such as Stemetil
- 5-HT3 receptor blockers, such as ondansetron (found in Zofran)
- H1 receptor blockers: antihistamines, such Benadryl and Phenergan; these are well known for travel sickness
- Cannabinoids (marijuana): mainstream medicine has a grudging and varied tolerance of this class of drugs for nausea from cancer treatments and other medical conditions.
- Benzodiazepines, such as Valium: these have a

demonstrable benefit for nausea and vomiting after
anaesthesia.

- Anti-cholinergics: these drugs are used to block the
autonomic nervous system by inhibiting one of its
neurotransmitters, acetylcholine. Some that you may
have heard of are Dramamine, commonly used for
motion sickness, and hyoscine (scopolamine), used in
anaesthesia or for travel sickness (as Kwells).

- Steroids, such as Dexamethasone: useful to prevent
the nausea associated with anaesthesia, but the way it
does so is not fully understood.

Triptans

Few drugs have been released with as much fanfare as the
triptans (key ingredients in the brand Sumatriptan) in the
early 1990s. These drugs were to be used for migraine and
cluster headaches, and the pre-release marketing was
impressive. The ads seemed to promise that migraine would
soon be a thing of the past; they included claims such as 'The
end of the headache that has lasted 2000 years' (a reference,
no doubt, to Cleopatra, one of history's more illustrious
migraineurs). The stumbling block was expense, but for
many, the price seemed be worth paying.

These medications have a similar effect to ergot
medications: they are selective serotonin receptor agonists.
For our purposes, 5-HT is synonymous with serotonin because
it is the precursor molecule. (For more on 5-HT, see Chapter
13.) The thinking of the original researchers went like this:
5-HT, ergotamine, and nor-adrenalin can all cause

vasoconstriction and relieve migraine attacks. Also, it was found, levels of 5-HT in platelets during a migraine attack are lowered. It was reasonable to assume, therefore, that low levels of serotonin were part of the pathology of migraine. 5-HT itself had too many side effects to be used as a drug, but 5-HT 'lookalikes' might just do the trick.

As it turned out, there were several types of 5-HT receptors, and some of these, when activated, actually cause blood vessels to dilate rather than constrict. So the aim was to find drugs that targeted the correct receptor. The original drug, Sumatriptan, was found to bind to a receptor named 5-HT 1D. Some newer drugs bind to 5-HT 1B/1D, and the drug Eletriptan binds to 1B/1D and 1F receptors.[109] Most of these receptors are located in the trigeminal nerve in the central nervous system. This fits in with the pivotal role that the trigeminal nerve plays in migraine and other headaches.

Then problems began to emerge. Some people found that taking the medication stopped the headache — only for it to reappear a few hours later. Warnings were issued about giving it to people with ischaemic heart disease or renal disease, or who had previously suffered from cerebrovascular disease. Doctors were not to prescribe it for use it within hours of ergot drugs. And we had to be on the lookout for serotonergic syndrome — the potentially dangerous condition caused by an overdose of serotonin (see Chapter 13). Some people developed altered heart rhythms such as bradycardia (slow heart rate) or tachycardia (rapid heart rate). Even seizures were reported. Some neurology clinics were said to be discouraged from using Sumatriptan.

Many people have taken this medication successfully, and

it has become the main treatment for some, but I find it hard to dismiss the risks. How do I know that my patient doesn't have silent heart disease? Certainly if I prescribe it and something goes wrong, the pharmaceutical industry is unlikely to rush to my defence. 'We did warn you' is about as much as I could expect. So another headache wonder pill has found me less than enthusiastic.

Strong analgesics or opioids

Elsewhere I have commented that sometimes the only humane treatment for a severe migraine attack (or cluster headache) is the use of an opiate, such as pethidine. This practice is generally frowned on, and is actively discouraged in emergency departments. This is easy to understand: migraine is a recurring illness, and dependence on opiates is a real risk. In the emergency room, where the doctor and patient don't know each other, drug addicts do feign migraine to get opiates.

However, for the family doctor, who knows the patient and is doing proper interim management, the use of pethidine seems both humane and appropriate. Those who rule against its use have, in all probability, never had a migraine. Yet even within a family practice, the risk of rebound headaches and dependence must be borne in mind constantly.

Drugs for prevention

Many patients have so many headaches that they need preventive treatment. Although my own approach is best represented in Chapter 8, let us look at the various medications in use.

Angiotensin II receptor antagonist

This family of drugs is used primarily for hypertension, but because they work by relaxing blood vessels, they also have some effect in preventing migraine attacks. The side effects include dizziness and potentially serious potassium retention. Candesartan is a commonly used member of this family of drugs.

Antidepressants

Old-fashioned tricyclic antidepressants, such as amitriptyline, have been noted to help reduce migraine attacks. This is thought to be independent of their actual antidepressant effect; rather, it is because they block the re-uptake of biogenic amines, such as serotonin and norepinephrine. In other words, they are having a serotonin agonist effect. More recently, it has been suggested that they also alter the sensitivity of dopaminergic receptors, with similar beneficial results on headaches.

Tricyclic anti-depressants can also have nasty side effects, especially on the heart — too high a dosage can cause cardiac arrhythmia — and can even cause toxicity. However, at the low doses used in migraine prevention, this is unlikely to be a significant problem.

Anti-epileptics

Some drugs in this class of medications have been used for migraine prophylaxis. Topiramate, Gabapentin, sodium valproate (an ingredient in brands such as Epilim), and valproic acid are among them. Yet an impressive list of side effects of these drugs raises the question of risks, and cost versus benefit.

Topiramate has been shown to have some effect in preventing migraines. Its downsides include abdominal pain, nausea, impaired concentration, speech difficulties, mood swings, visual disturbances and nystagmus (uncontrolled rapid eye movements), kidney stones, and weight loss. Even psychotic symptoms have been reported.

Sodium valproate, an anti-convulsant, has also been used as a mood stabiliser and a migraine prophylactic. Side effects include weight gain, dyspepsia, birth defects, and a risk of subsequent autism in the foetus.

Antihistamines

A commonly used 'preventer' is pizotifen, the key ingredient in the drug Sandomigran. It is prescribed for vascular headaches, cluster headaches, and the various types of migraine. It is an antihistamine, and actually works as a serotonin antagonist on 5-HT 1 and 5-HT 2A receptors. The side effects include weight gain and drowsiness. Many find it helpful, although I am not convinced that it does much to hold severe recurrent headache at bay.

Cyproheptadine, the key ingredient in the drug Periactin (or Peritol), is an antihistamine that also acts as a 5-HT 2 receptor antagonist; it is therefore anti-serotonergic. It is also a calcium channel blocker, and so may help those whose headache genes are linked to calcium channel disorders (discussed shortly).

Beta blockers

These drugs are named for the fact that they block the actions of adrenalin by attaching to one group of adrenalin receptors, the beta receptors. The receptors are in the central nervous system, and as adrenalin is a significant neurotransmitter, such an inhibition can be helpful. Although many patients say that they get their headaches only when they are stressed, in Chapter 1 we mentioned the classic 'Friday-night headache', which occurs when the stress comes off and relaxation, somewhat paradoxically, leads to headache. This shows just how complex the action of neurotransmitters can be.

Several factors limit the use of beta blockers. The most important is that they affect the adrenergic receptors that operate throughout the body, including heart, lungs, blood vessels, liver, and pancreas. The term 'adrenergic' means 'acting like adrenalin'. Adrenergic receptors that predominate in the cardiovascular system are referred to as beta-1 receptors, and those mostly found in the bronchioles of the lung are beta-2 receptors. Some beta-blocking drugs are selective in their activity (such as 'cardioselective' medications, which work on the heart), but some affect *all* receptors.

Because of the potential for risky side effects — namely, producing in the heart or lungs the very opposite effect to the one you want — it is generally thought wise for asthmatics and those with certain heart conditions to avoid beta blockers. There is a worrying list of drug interactions between beta blockers and a range of medications, including some types of blood pressure pills, antidepressants, antibiotics, and antihistamines.

Having said this, the beta blockers propranolol, metoprolol, and timolol are all used at times as migraine preventers.

Botulinum toxin (botox)

This medication is in a class all of its own. Botulin is a neurotoxic poison, but it can be very effective in some cases. It is expensive because it has to be injected by an experienced doctor at repeated intervals, and because the drug itself is costly. However, 'miracle cures' are sometimes talked about, and this is incorrect. The drug only lasts about six months before another injection is needed.

Botulinum toxin has been used in treating migraine, sometimes with considerable benefit.[110] There are also reports of success in cluster headaches, tension headache, and the management of chronic daily headache.[111] Patients interested in trying this treatment should consult with a neurologist.

Calcium channel blockers

We have seen that antihistamines such as Periactin operate to block calcium channels. This is significant when we consider how many of the genes involved in migraine affect the calcium channels. Also relevant are the other genetic determinants of migraine, and the effectiveness of magnesium in migraine management (see Chapter 8). Magnesium has often been described as nature's calcium channel blocker. Once again, I make the point that the modern Western diet is lacking in magnesium.

Having said that, Verapamil, a calcium channel blocker used primarily for hypertension and heart disease, has found its place for migraine prevention. It is also sometimes used for the prevention of cluster headaches, paroxysmal hemicrania, and the group of headaches referred to as the 'trigeminal autonomic cephalalgias'. Side effects include dizziness and fatigue.

Methysergide

Again, this drug is in a class of its own. It is a semi-synthetic ergot alkaloid. It acts as a serotonin receptor antagonist, working on the 5-HT 2 receptors. Its use has been to prevent severe and recurrent migraine and cluster headaches.

Methysergide has nasty side effects of retroperitoneal, pleural, and heart-valve fibrosis (described by one of my lecturers as setting these tissues in cement), which have led British authorities to advise against its use, except under hospital supervision. It is not a medication that I would ever be comfortable to prescribe. Although it is said to be one of the most effective drugs of all, I have seen patients whose response does not, in my mind, warrant the risks involved in using it.

Oestrogen

Oestrogen, usually applied as a gel, is sometimes used for 'menstrual migraine'. It is another medication that I am uncomfortable with. However, quite a few women, having been given it by another doctor, request repeat scripts from me because they have found it helpful.

Alpha-2 adrenergic agonist

This drug is rarely used, and is included only to make this list complete. Beta blockers (discussed on page 214) are more commonly used for migraine than this class of drug.

Its name refers to the receptors for adrenalin, which has both alpha and beta receptors. Clonidine (the key ingredient in the drug Dixarit) is an alpha-2 agonist, and is sometimes used as a migraine prophylactic. It has the side effects of dry mouth, dizziness, and constipation. The British National

Formulary lists side effects such as nausea, cardiac arrhythmias, depression, and insomnia as reasons for cautioning against its use. It is still used in Australia, but very rarely.

Disadvantages of drugs for prevention

Looking at these impressive lists of drugs for headaches, I am reminded of the words of one of my lecturers, four decades ago, in medical school. He said that the longer the list of treatments for any condition, the more likely it is that none of them are much good — otherwise you wouldn't have to keeping finding more.

Many of these medications are intended to be either/or treatments. That is not to suggest that headache clinics routinely advise the taking of several medications at any one time. However, some *are* used in combination or in sequence when first-line treatment has not alleviated the headache, and the person goes to the next drug on a list. Many patients that I see have, in desperation, combined the medications in an alarming manner. Side effects can be unpleasant, or even life threatening, when inappropriate combinations are used. Ironically, headache is a known side effect of some of them.

Medication is a crutch and, like all crutches, has its place. But we do well to remember that much headache research is driven by drug companies seeking profit. Under new conventions for declaration of conflict of interest, the neurologist author of a recent article on headaches I read in a journal for GPs admitted his connections: he had acted as a consultant to two different pharmaceutical companies, and received speaker fees from both. This is not an unusual situation.

PART III
The Science Behind Headache

This section should be read as a glossary or reference by those who want more detail. It is not essential for managing your headaches.

CHAPTER 10
The Biological Basis: types of headache and their link to genes

'A wise man should consider that health is the greatest of human blessings, and learn how by his own thought to derive benefit from his illnesses.'
HIPPOCRATES

We start this chapter with a closer look at the classification of the various types of headaches. The list, as drawn up by the International Headache Society, is still just a fraction of the total, but it covers the main categories seen in clinical practice. The remainder of the chapter will give more insight into the genetic factors influencing these various types of headache.

CLASSIFICATION OF HEADACHES

As we work our ways through the various types of headache, we see the problems faced by the International Headache

Society when they embarked on the mammoth task of trying to classify headache. Some headaches have historically been grouped by symptoms, and others by suspected causative factors, such as histamine. There is a lot of overlap in many headaches. Sometimes one outstanding symptom has given the headache its name, as with ice-pick and thunderclap headaches, which may in fact occur across a range of headache types.

Cluster headache

Cluster headache is nicknamed 'the suicide headache'. It affects about 0.1 per cent of the population and occurs mostly in men. The pain far outstrips that of even the most severe migraine, and has been described as the worst a human can experience. Frequent sufferers have considered many desperate solutions, hence the nickname.

The pain can last from 15 minutes to upwards of three hours, and one attack can follow within minutes of the previous one. Attack-free periods can last months or years, which gives rise to the term 'cluster'.

Doctor Peter Goadsby, the Australian specialist mentioned in Chapter 5, is one of the researchers who trace the problem to the hypothalamus. One reason is that these headaches tend to occur with a diurnal or seasonal pattern, and the hypothalamus is a control centre for our biological clocks. So this is where magic mushrooms, mentioned in Chapter 8, fit in. If drugs such as LSD and psilocybin can dampen down the activity in the hypothalamus, maybe we can learn more about cluster headache, while offering some relief to its victims.[112]

I remember a neurosurgeon lamenting that he was one of

the few people around who could not get hold of heroin. A drug that had left a patient lucid while treating their intractable cancer pain was available to every addict on the street, but was denied to him, on threat of loss of registration, if he wanted to use it therapeutically. Will this be the fate of LSD if it proves to be a viable treatment for the suicide headache?

Family pedigrees indicate a genetic component in cluster headaches, as discussed in Chapter 2. Food associations and triggers (discussed in Chapters 3 and 4) also play a role. The separation of bullets from triggers is somewhat arbitrary. But in summary, 'bullet' foods for this type of headache include chocolate and bananas, along with foods high in nitrites, such as bacon and preserved meats. Triggers include smoking, alcohol, MSG, hydrocarbons (from petroleum solvents and from perfume), orgasm, and the drug glyceryl trinitrate (used to treat angina).

These headaches are often known as 'histamine headaches' — although this term is sometimes also used of migraine. Management of these headaches has involved avoiding foods that contain or release histamine.

Medication-overuse headache

This heading is added for completeness. It can apply to any headache, and the original symptoms can be exaggerated as the 'need' for the medication becomes the dominant feature. Relevant aspects are covered under 'chronic daily headache' below.

Migraine

Migraine affects about 18 per cent of women and 8 per cent of men, although some estimates have the figure as high as one in four of the population as a whole.[113] One has to wonder whether the uncertainty is due to a diagnostic difficulty or to an upward shift in the incidence. Migraines are divided into two groups: migraine with aura (MA), which occurs in about 25 per cent of migraineurs, and migraine without aura (MO, or common migraine), which occurs in about 75 per cent. Key features of both types of migraine are pain (typically confined to one side of the head) and vomiting. Also common is a sense of disorientation, and sensitivity to bright light or glare. However, every headache is different, and not all features are present from headache to headache, even in the same patient. I often find myself listening to an individual who, to my ears, is clearly describing a migraine. But they will say that their headaches are not migrainous because they are missing one feature from the menu of migraine symptoms that they read on Wikipedia, or found in a textbook somewhere.

Migraine with aura (MA)

This is typically a severe headache, usually on one side of the head. It affects about 12 per cent of the female population and only 6 per cent of males. As a result, hormonal factors are thought to be involved.

The headache is often preceded by warning signs, known as an aura. Auras can take the form of flashing lights or jagged lines. Sometimes there is temporary loss of vision in the visual field of one eye. Some people report dysphoria — a sense of altered reality. It is this sense of dysphoria that has led to the belief that Vincent van Gogh's art and Lewis Carroll's imagination were inspired by migraine auras.

When the headache hits, there is often extreme sensitivity to light and sound, and nausea and vomiting are a feature. Migraine with aura can last from four to 72 hours. The most common theory of what is happening at a biochemical level is that an alteration in the serotonergic system leads to a 'migraine cascade', a series of events that lead to a migraine.

This type of headache is known to be associated with stroke, so the use of hormone therapy in these patients is thought to be very risky. Variants of MA include sporadic hemiplegic migraine and familial hemiplegic migraine (see Chapter 2 and below).

Familial hemiplegic migraine

This headache is a type of MA, with added worrying features. The clinical picture is one of weakness down one side of the body and sometimes ataxia (a staggering gait), seizures, or even coma.

The headache itself is of the 'classic' variety, with aura, nausea, and severe pain. The presentation can look like a stroke — and indeed, stroke is a real risk.

There are three clinical sub-types of familial hemiplegic migraine, each based on the associated gene. These will be discussed shortly (under 'More about genes').

Migraine-associated vertigo (MAV)

Migraine associated with vertigo is generally classified into three groups.

- **Vestibular migraine:** This term is used to describe a migrainous headache when the pathology seems to be centred on the part of the inner ear known as the vestibule. The symptoms include dizziness, vertigo, and extreme sensitivity to motion. Individuals may also experience muffled hearing and tinnitus (ringing in the affected ear).
- **Basilar migraine:** This is the most dramatic form of MAV, wherein the individual also develops symptoms of brainstem or occipital lobe dysfunction. These include hearing impairment, slurred speech, temporary loss of sight, and temporary loss of consciousness. Because of such frightening aspects, medical intervention may be required to distinguish the symptoms from stroke.
- **Vertiginous migraine:** Many people experience giddiness during a migraine, often as part of the aura.

In each of these three headaches, vertigo is a marked feature. Yet if the criteria of the International Headache Society are used, in some of these cases it is not possible to make a diagnosis of migraine at all.

Migraine without aura (MO, or common migraine)

MO has many of the features of MA but, as the name states, it lacks the aura. Clinically, the presentation is often less severe, with the sufferer sometimes able to (heroically) battle through a normal day's work. As we have seen in Chapter 2, the genetics appear to be different from MA. It is not uncommon to see both kinds of headache present in the one person at different times. Such individuals may have more than one set of predisposing genes, and may be subject to similar triggers for both types of headache.

Abdominal migraine (cyclic vomiting in children)

Abdominal migraine is far from unusual. In fact, in children it is one of the most common presentations of migraine. I include it here because it is so often missed. A child who complains of a sore tummy, or goes through bouts of vomiting for which there is no obvious cause, is often suffering from 'atypical' migraine. They do not usually complain of headaches — though when questioned, will sometimes admit to them.

It is hard to categorise the *type* of headache this pain may eventually turn into. The general belief is that migraine is often so undifferentiated in children that we have to look at it differently; we need to ask, 'Could this be early migraine?' Family history can help in determining the presence of migraine. It should also be remembered that even very young children can exhibit symptoms similar to those of adults. Some will maintain this 'abdominal' form of migraine throughout life.

Ice-pick headache

This graphic term describes a type of headache that seems to occur as sudden, discrete stabbing pains behind the eyes or in the head, especially in the temporal region. The logic of the name is immediately apparent to patients who have experienced this kind of pain. It is also sometimes called 'primary stabbing headache'.

The pain typically lasts for five to 30 seconds, but may be repeated throughout the day. It is seen most commonly in those patients we would describe as migraineurs, although it has also been used to describe cluster-headache pain. However, unlike migraine, these attacks usually occur without aura, dysphoria, nausea, or vomiting and, in contrast to cluster headache, their brief duration usually renders them comparatively tolerable. Melatonin, magnesium, vitamin B2, and CoQ10 (see Chapter 8) are said to be useful in the management of attacks.

Paroxysmal hemicrania

The rare headache known as paroxysmal hemicrania is easy to confuse with either migraine or cluster headaches. The diagnosis is usually made by neurologists, who regard it as separate from migraine. It occurs in intense bouts that last from minutes to more than half an hour. The pain is severe; it is confined to one side of the head, and often accompanied by weeping of the eye and swelling of the eyelid on that side. The pain is described as 'boring' or 'throbbing'. The headaches may occur daily for something like a year, and then disappear for months, or even years; or they may occur sporadically. Certain neck movements can set them off, as can glyceryl trinitrate, a medication used for angina.

The US National Institute of Neurological Disorders and Stroke has undertaken research into the causes and management of this headache. Treatments include NSAIDs, calcium channel blockers, and steroids.

Tension headache

Tension headache is regarded as the most common type, accounting for about 90 per cent of all headache presentation. Incidence varies from population to population.

In contrast to migraine, the pain in tension headache is not confined to one side of the head; it occurs at the back of the neck, across the forehead, or on the top of the head. The pain, which is often described as like a band or, in more severe cases, a vice, is usually accompanied by a stiff neck. It can be mild to moderate in intensity, and may respond to simple interventions such as rest or meditation. Generally, the more frequent the headache, the more severe the pain.

Poor posture, jaw clenching, and dental and neck problems are often considered triggers of this type of headache.

The biochemistry is thought to include the serotonergic neurotransmitters, as it does with migraine. Analgesics such as aspirin and paracetamol are not highly effective, but tricyclic antidepressants seem to have some benefit. Other medications that act on the serotonergic pathways, such as SSRIs, are often prescribed, but their use is not supported by clinical studies. Headaches that respond to small doses of alcohol or the benzodiazepams seem to fit the tension headache profile — but these drugs are poor choices for treatment!

There are three sub-groups of this type of headache.

- **Tension-type headache (TTH):** This occurs periodically, and is readily relieved with simple interventions such as rest or meditation.
- **Episodic tension-type headache (ETTH):** This is deemed to be present when the headache occurs at

least twice a week but on less than 15 days in a month.

- **Chronic tension-type headache (CTTH):** In 2004, the International Headache Society deemed that to be classified as 'chronic', the headache needed to occur on more than 15 days per month over a minimum period of six months.

Clinically, any of the tension headaches can be difficult to distinguish from migraine, even though they are not usually unilateral.

Chronic daily headache (CDH)

The term chronic daily headache, introduced by the International Headache Society in 2004, refers to one sort of chronic tension-type headache. It was coined to cover those patients whose history precluded neat inclusion into categories like 'tension headache' or 'migraine', and the term now covers any headache where the most salient feature is frequency and persistence. The subgroups involve chronic tension-type, chronic, or 'transformed' migraine, medication-overuse headache, cluster headache, and the interestingly named 'hemicrania continua'.

All doctors treating headaches have these patients — and they provide the biggest challenges of all.[114] In CDH, we see the greatest convergence of headache pathology, and perhaps this is where the most lessons are to be learned. For this reason, I will devote some space to this headache, going beyond the classification — or 'naming the bird', in Feynman's terms — to look at the bird itself more closely.

CDH: a narrative

There are a couple of reasons why this headache is interesting. First, it explodes the idea that headaches can be boxed neatly into a rigid classification. Second, with an estimated incidence of 2–8 per cent of the entire population, these people include some of the most desperate patients of all. In all the treatment guidelines, the message is clear: get the patient's pain under control (usually, it is assumed, by means of medication) or the headaches will become harder to treat. The implication is that some process occurring during the various headaches leads to irreversible damage.

To explain this, it is easy to invoke any of the theories discussed in Chapter 5: vascular, neuronal dysfunction, or damage inflicted by inflammatory cytokines.

Let's look at some of the characteristics of CDH. Especially when the primary headache has been migrainous, the phenomenon known as allodynia is often seen. The patient reacts to a simple stimulus — light touch or pressure, or a mild temperature change — with an exaggerated pain response. The related but separate condition known as hyperacusis (intolerance to everyday sounds as if they were painful) was discussed in Chapter 7. The neurons in the pain pathway have become sensitised, so that they now seem to be wired up to fire at much lower thresholds.

What is going on here? The answer is not certain. Sensitisation of NMDA receptors (mentioned in Chapter 13) is certainly involved. But we also know that in CDH, iron is deposited in the brain. One of the main areas for this is the part of the midbrain known as the periaquaductal grey matter, or PAG, area. A detailed discussion of the PAG area appears in Chapter 11, but basically, this area of the brain is thought to be central to all headaches. Iron deposition may either be marker or a contributing factor to what is now thought of as low-grade brain damage associated with CDH. MRI studies have supported this finding both in migrainous CDH and in CDH that has been shown to be due to medication overuse. The implication is that iron deposits have something to do with the perpetuation of the headaches, as well as signalling low-grade brain damage. (For more on long-term effects of headache, see 'white matter lesions' in Chapter 12.) Hence the motivation to get the patient's headaches under control. The important question is: how can this be done?

Thunderclap headache

This has nothing to do with the weather headache discussed in Chapter 4. It is named for its dramatic onset, so sudden that the victim feels as if they have been struck over the head.

Thunderclap headache can be part of the spectrum of tension headache, migraine, cluster headache, or cough headache. But this sudden pain may be more sinister: it can be the result of a cerebrovascular accident such as thrombosis, haemorrhage, or stroke. A rare cause is an odd tumour known as a phaeochromocytoma, which releases sporadic bursts of adrenalin. Such headaches warrant urgent medical attention.

Trigeminal autonomic cephalalgias and atypical facial pain

Just in case we were settling into the idea that headaches are mostly migrainous, tension-type, chronic daily, or medication-overuse, along comes another set of headaches to make classification harder. There is always one patient who complains of head and neck pain that does not seem to fit into any of the common classifications. Such people often return from a consultation with a neurologist having been diagnosed with one of a whole miscellany of head and neck pain. These are a group of odd and relatively rare 'neuralgias', usually diagnosed by a neurologist. The pain can be fierce, sometimes quite localised, and cause much anxiety for the sufferer.

Trigeminal neuralgia

Although not strictly speaking a 'headache', this exquisitely painful condition raises questions about the nature and causes of head and neck pain. Trigeminal neuralgia is classified as either typical or atypical.

- The typical form causes electric-like shocks in the region of the face, teeth, and jaw. These attacks last from seconds to minutes, and can lead to adverse psychosocial effects. They are usually treated with the anti-convulsant carbamazepine.
- The atypical variant can last longer, and persistent pain is its distinguishing characteristic. The antidepressant amitriptyline is the first-line treatment for this, but a range of other medications, from anti-convulsants through to gabapentin (a drug that mimics the neurotransmitter gamma-aminobutyric acid, or GABA), are employed.

Further discussion of these types of head pain are beyond the scope of this book.

MORE ABOUT GENES

In Chapter 2, we looked briefly at genes associated with the more common types of headache, which can be helped by simple nutritional approaches. Let's now look at the genetic detail in relation to some less common headaches.

An understanding of genetics in any area of medicine is only useful if we can use it to improve prevention and treatment. Because it is clear that headache can be linked with diet and lifestyle, any clues to modifications we can make will be valuable. As you read on, you may think that you do not get the type of headache we discuss, but if some of the symptoms sound like yours, be open to the possibility that you may. Not all people with vulnerable genes get the worst-case outcome; often they may get a much milder form. So let us look at some genes.

Familial hemiplegic migraine (FHM) genes

It was a rare form of headache, familial hemiplegic migraine, that first lent weight to the idea that headache could have a hereditary basis. Eventually, three genes for FHM were identified and named for the condition.

- **FHM1 (CACNA1A):** This gene, located on chromosome 19, affects membrane structures known as 'calcium channels'. More than a dozen gene variants produce the defect responsible for FHM1. Some of the variants of this gene have an undesirable effect on the release of neurotransmitters, which helps explain sensitivity to noise and light, and probably sensitivity to fumes, in some sufferers.

- **FHM2 (ATP1A2):** This gene is found on chromosome 1 and is responsible for an enzyme that works to maintain the balance between sodium and potassium in the body. The gene is particularly active in the astrocytes of the brain. (The function of astrocytes, and their role in headaches, is discussed in Chapter 11.)
- **FHM3 (SCN1A):** This gene, located on chromosome 2, affects a sodium channel. The comments just made apply equally here.

Chapter 13 suggests that certain headaches are manifestations of 'ion channelopathies', a growing area of medical research. All three variants of FHM could be classed as ion channelopathies. These genes determine how the body handles simple nutrients such as calcium, magnesium, potassium, and sodium.

As we saw in Chapter 8, the modern diet does not preserve nature's balance between calcium and magnesium, and it actually reverses the ratio of sodium to potassium from that which is found in the hunter-gatherer diet. The balance among these nutrients is vital, and getting it right could lead to interventions that are safer, and possibly better, than many of the medications we currently use.

In the case of a calcium channelopathy, the problem may be a relative overload of calcium in relation to magnesium intake. Modern agriculture tips the balance in favour of calcium.

The role of magnesium as a headache treatment is discussed in Chapter 8.

Other genes

Many doctors who see headache patients on a regular basis find that several of them link their headaches to direct environmental inputs, such as dietary factors and chemical exposure of various kinds. Our genetic makeup determines how our body handles these challenges, and so genes are directly relevant to headache. In fact, we are at the dawn of an era in which gene testing will become central to most health problems.

Detailed examination of many other sorts of genes is beyond the scope of this book, but in Chapter 12 we will have a closer look at some genes associated with the ability to detoxify common noxious chemicals. First, however, let's look briefly at a couple of other important genes.

- **GAD genes.** These are the genes that code for the enzyme glutamic acid decarboxylase. This enzyme is responsible for converting glutamate to a calming neurotransmitter, GABA. An inability to do this allows glutamate to go towards stimulation of micro-glial cells, causing agitation and headache. (This is shown in Diagram 1 on page 50.) The GAD genes are polymorphic, and some of us were luckier than others in the ones we inherited.

  GABA has been targeted by medication, notably the anti-epileptic drug gabapentin, and some herbals such as valerian and gotu kola. Self-medication is not advised, but avoiding MSG is.

- **Genes associated with vitamin D status.** All we will say on this topic is that migraine, tension headaches, and chronic pain syndromes have been linked to genes associated with vitamin D status, and we can assume that such genes also play a part in headache susceptibility.

- **MHC genes, also known as HLA genes or 'major histocompatibility complex' genes.** They were discussed briefly in Chapter 6 and are a clue to our genetic (and geographic) origins. The possibility exists that they determine the kind of foods most suitable for us, based on what was available to our ancestors. These genes will not be discussed further in this book.
- **NOS genes.** These genes determine our ability to make the enzyme nitric oxide synthetase, which will be discussed in detail in Chapter 13. The point to make here is that, like GAD genes, these genes are polymorphic, and our draw in this genetic lottery is yet another significant player in terms of headache risk.

TOXICITY AND DETOXIFICATION

In this chapter and in Chapter 12, we meet some of the enzymes that help us to deal with substances such as sulphur, and the genetic factors that explain why some people are made sicker by sulphur derivatives than others. Here, we also look at some other genes that determine how different individuals deal with certain chemicals.

It may seem strange that such genes are not studied in the

context of headache. I think that this is because the role of toxins in health generally, and headache specifically, has been seriously overlooked by doctors.

Toxicity and the liver

Chapter 3 looked at the various ways in which our immune system might react to a food and lead on to a headache. But we also saw that our adverse reaction may have nothing to do with our immune system, but may be a response to some chemical component of the food we eat. We also saw that all our food, healthy or otherwise, contains such chemicals.

We each have a liver in order to deal with these chemicals. The liver processes food so that it is more likely to nourish us than to make us sick. It is there to protect us from the poisons that occur in nature, and nowadays it also has to deal with chemicals that come out of the factory.

The liver works by means of enzymes, and some livers are better at it than others. I emphasise that the same enzymes get pressed into service to process not only foods, but also drug-like foods, such as coffee and alcohol; recreational drugs; the drugs that you buy over the counter, such as aspirin, paracetamol, and non-steroidal anti-inflammatory drugs; the drugs that your doctor gives you a prescription for; and also the household or agricultural chemicals that come your way from any source.

The idea of 'toxicity' can be anthropocentric. From nature's point of view, molecules are not just 'good' and 'bad'. Certain chemicals are almost always toxic, but sometimes it's a question of balance between 'currently needed' and 'currently not needed'. Some of us are better at detoxing chemicals than others. Not surprisingly, the reason for this is, in part at least, under genetic control.

Biotransformation

When the liver encounters something that is potentially toxic or out of balance, it deals with it by a process known as 'biotransformation'. It does this to maintain our hormone levels, for example.

There are four kinds of biotransformation reactions: oxidation, reduction, degradation, conjugation. Most of them are carried out by enzymes, which are classified as phase-1 enzymes, phase-2 enzymes, and mixed-function enzymes.

Phase-1 enzymes

Phase-1 enzymes account for the first three of the processes in the list above: oxidation, reduction, and degradation.

The multi-gene cytochrome P450 system is a superfamily of enzymes and is responsible for a large number of phase-1 reactions. Often abbreviated to CYP, its enzymes have been found in plants, animals, fungi, and even viruses. It carries out oxidation, reduction, and degradation. It plays an important role in both the synthesis and the breakdown of hormones such as oestrogen and testosterone, vitamin D, cholesterol, and even bile. Many drugs are detoxified by these enzymes.

Phase-2 enzymes

Phase-2 enzymes are responsible for conjugation. This biotransformation or detoxification occurs when the enzyme sticks another molecule onto the 'toxin'.

Conjugation reactions facilitated by phase-2 enzymes are classified into various groups, such as 'glucuronidation', 'acetylation', 'glycination', and 'sulphation'. To take the first of these: our liver 'glucuronidates' oestrogen when it decides that we have too much and need to get rid of some. Pesticides and plastics that degrade to oestrogen-like molecules can interfere with this process by overloading the system.

Some phase-1 genes

The effectiveness of any of our enzymes will be determined by the gene we inherited for that enzyme. Let us look at some known weak spots.

Oxidation (hydroxylation)

Hydroxylation is one of the means by which oxidation of a chemical can occur. The CYP enzymes use hydroxylation as a means to detoxify some chemicals. Caffeine is one such chemical, and the first phase of its metabolism is performed in the liver. Withdrawal symptoms frequently occur when the drugs and chemicals that are metabolised by these CYP enzymes are withheld, so the phenomenon of caffeine withdrawal should come as no surprise to us.

Caffeine is a good example of the way in which our individual genetic makeup affects our response to a food or drug. While some people seem to be able to sleep after strong coffee, others find that small amounts cause insomnia and can set off palpitations or even headaches.

About 9 per cent of the British population are known to be slow hydroxylators because they have certain polymorphisms in their genetic makeup that affect the CYP enzymes. However, the British researcher Jean Monro was able to show that as many as 66 per cent of chemically sensitive people had this genotype.[115] So if you find that you react to small doses of coffee, and easily get sick from chemicals of various kinds, you are probably a slow hydroxylator.

Genes for sulphite oxidase (SUOX)

In Chapter 13, we look at a genetic weakness that affects this particular phase-1 enzyme. We will see how a vulnerable polymorphism may make people more sensitive to sulphur drugs and sulphurous gases.

Genes for monoamine oxidase (MAO)

Not all phase-1 enzymes are from the CYP family. This gene and diamine oxidase code for important non-CYP enzymes.

Chapters 4 and 13 look at a range of chemicals that are amines of one sort or another. Some, such as serotonin, melatonin, epinephrine, and dopamine, are well-known neurotransmitters; others are to be found in our food.

The body uses both phase-1 and phase-2 enzymes to metabolise amines. This phase-1 enzyme comes in two forms: MAO A and MAO B. The first works mainly on the catecholamines (a type of neurotransmitter) and serotonin. Both work on tyramine, tryptamine, and serotonin.

The genes that help us make MAO are non-CYP genes. They are polymorphic, and research on the contribution of different SNiPs seems to indicate an increased risk of migraine with some variants.

Gene for diamine oxidase (DAO)

Diamine oxidase is an enzyme that carries out biotransformation by oxidation, and it does not belong to the CYP family either. Genetically, some people have a deficiency in this enzyme, which means that they have trouble breaking down the histamine they make (or eat).

We know that histamine headaches are often associated with alcohol. Alcohol liberates histamine from body stores, and people who are low in diamine oxidase are slower at breaking down this histamine. Things may be even worse if they are also iodine-deficient because, as we shall see in Chapter 13, they may be turning more of their dietary histidine into histamine.

Some phase-2 genes

Once the liver has finished processing a molecule with its phase-1 enzymes, it starts using phase-2 enzymes. Again, our ability to do this depends on the phase-2 genes that we have inherited.

Acetylation genes

Several genes control acetylation reactions, and two types of acetylation reaction are relevant here.

First, acetylation is one way in which the body approaches a toxic chemical. It can use an enzyme to acetylate it, which helps the body to get rid of the chemical by making it more soluble. Up to half the population of Europe are thought to be slow acetylators, so this is hardly a defect. However, if you are of this genotype, you have an increased risk of auto-immune disease, and of bad reactions to chemicals and drugs.

The second area where acetylation genes matter is in relation to our DNA. The genes involved are histone acetyl transferase and histone deacetyalse. You really don't need to know more than that they help to determine when and where our *other* genes are read.

Genes for phenolsulphotransferase

Sulphur is an important element in human chemistry, but also a source of considerable confusion once the question of 'sulphur allergy' arises. This topic is discussed in some detail in Chapter 13, where we look at how the body deals with sulphur and some other phase-2 enzymes, the sulpho-transferases.

The genetic information we have just been looking at is unlikely to help you manage your day-to-day headache at the moment. But in the future, I think it will help to unravel the answers to questions like 'Why me?', 'What about my family?', and 'Why does this drug help some people and not me?' And importantly, it may help to answer the questions of what causes headache and which actions different individuals should take to prevent them.

CHAPTER 11

Headache Anatomy: where and why they start

'Anatomy is destiny.'
SIGMUND FREUD

I do not agree with Freud. It's true that your anatomy — if you are tall or short, attractive or plain, and certainly if you are male or female — will have a big impact on the life you will lead. In terms of your health, however, my vote would go to the slogan 'genes are destiny'.

Still, there is a place for a discussion about the anatomy of headache, and that is what we will deal with in this chapter. Anatomy expresses itself through the nervous system, and the muscles, blood vessels, gastrointestinal tract, glands, and skin that support that nervous system. So we'd better familiarise ourselves with some terms in order to avoid misconceptions.

The six anatomical systems that we will look at in this chapter are:

- the nervous system
- the cardiovascular system

- the musculoskeletal system
- dentition
- the gastrointestinal system
- the endocrine system.

THE NERVOUS SYSTEM

Our nervous system is made up of is made up of two parts: the central and peripheral nervous systems (see Diagram 3). The central nervous system consists of the brain and the spinal cord. They communicate with the rest of the body through the peripheral nervous system. There are further subdivisions, which we will also look at.

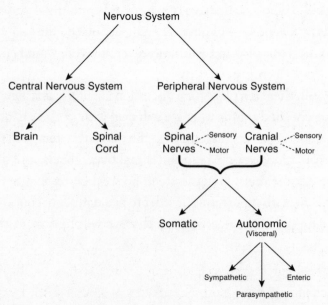

Diagram 3: the nervous system

The peripheral nervous system (PNS)

Let us start with the peripheral nervous system, which has two trunk lines — the incoming, or sensory, nervous system, and the outgoing, or motor, nervous system. All the messages coming into and going out of the brain are carried in these large trunk lines via the cranial and spinal nerves. The spinal nerves carry all their messages to the brain via the spinal cord; the cranial nerves go directly to the brain.

There are 12 cranial nerves, and in a fortunate vote for sanity, they are numbered I to XII. They also have descriptive names, such as 'trigeminal' and 'vagus', and we shall look at some of them presently.

The peripheral nervous system is further divided into the somatic parts and the visceral or autonomic parts. By and large, we have conscious control of what happens in the somatic arm of the nervous system, but the autonomic nervous system is generally beyond our conscious control. However, practitioners of Western medicine are slowly beginning to learn what traditions such as yoga and Ayurveda have made clear for a long time: practices of meditation and biofeedback can influence digestion, the stress response, blood pressure, and other such visceral functions.

Where autonomic function concerns the gut, it has been described as the 'second brain'. The presence in the gut of neurotransmitters found in the brain, such as serotonin and dopamine, reinforces this idea. The autonomic nervous system also has cells within in it that resemble the glial cells in the brain. Moreover, the gut seems to share a defence mechanism against 'non-self' substances, similar to the blood–brain barrier of the central nervous system. (This barrier marks out the blood vessels of the brain as different from the other blood vessels in our body. Tight junctions in their linings mean that only very small particles can get from the blood into the brain. This protects the brain from most bacteria and viruses, and from many chemicals.)

Most people find it easy to grasp the idea of a 'second brain'. Our language reflects this in expressions such as 'I have a gut feeling.' A migraineur experiencing the nausea of migraine before any head pain begins can identify the nausea as something connected to the impending headache, and quite different to that felt when they have eaten something bad, or eaten too much.

The autonomic nervous system was traditionally divided into the sympathetic and parasympathetic branches. In recent times, a third subdivision has been suggested — the enteric nervous system.

The neurotransmitters associated with the sympathetic nervous system are adrenalin and nor-adrenalin (also known as epinephrine and nor-epinephrine). In the parasympathetic system, the predominant neurotransmitter is acetylcholine. In Chapter 9, we learned about drugs used for headache that target these neurotransmitters.

- The **sympathetic nervous system** mobilises body systems for 'fight or flight'. Blood is directed away from the gut and skin, and redirected towards the muscles, lungs, and heart. Gut and urinary sphincters are constricted.

   Special features of the sympathetic nervous system include controlling our sweat glands, and connecting to the adrenal medulla (part of the adrenal gland) sitting on top of our kidneys, which is the source of the hormone adrenalin. Many people with headaches identify themselves as 'sympathetic dominant', meaning that they tend to be overanxious. People who experience 'white-coat hypertension' — whose blood pressure rises in the presence of a health practitioner — are activating their sympathetic nervous system, mostly quite contrary to their conscious wishes.

- The **parasympathetic nervous system** is activated when we are relaxing. Parasympathetic functions include promoting digestion, accommodating to close visual work, slowing the heart rate, and promoting sexual arousal. The parasympathetic nervous system uses the cranial nerves III, VII, IX, and X, and the spinal nerves S2, S3, and S4. Cranial nerve X, the vagus nerve, is of particular interest to headache sufferers. We will discuss this shortly.

- The **enteric nervous system** is associated with the gut and the lungs. This third classification has been proposed because the neurotransmitter involved may be nitric oxide, rather than either adrenalin or acetylcholine.

A healthy balance between the three branches of the autonomic nervous system is what practitioners of chiropractic and teachers of yoga and meditation are aiming for when they see headache sufferers. The curious yogic tradition of alternate nostril breathing is one example of an attempt to balance the sympathetic and parasympathetic nervous systems.

The central nervous system (CNS)

The central nervous system has many components, and quite a number of them are implicated in headaches. Here is a quick tour of the brain.

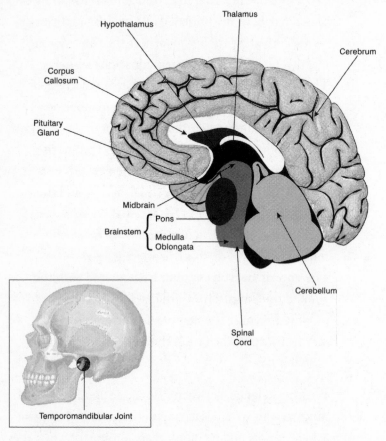

Diagram 4: the human brain

- **Cerebrum:** This is what most of us think about when we refer to our brain. The outer layer, known as the cerebral cortex, is where sensory information is received and processed. We sometimes refer to it as our 'grey matter' because of its colour; the inner part of the brain is known as the 'white matter'.
- **Cerebellum:** Known as the hindbrain, this is responsible for the coordination of movement, balance, and equilibrium.
- **Midbrain:** This sits immediately below the cerebrum. It links the cerebrum to the brainstem.
- **Brainstem:** The brainstem joins onto the spinal cord below it. It controls basic bodily functions such as breathing, swallowing, heart rate, and blood pressure; it is concerned with consciousness, and impacts on wakefulness. The brainstem begins with the pons, which relays sensory information between the cerebrum and the cerebellum. The lower half of the brainstem contains the medulla, which helps to control the brainstem's autonomic functions and also contains the vomiting and vasomotor centres. The function of the latter is to control blood pressure by coordinating the heart rate and blood-vessel diameter.
- **Hypothalamus:** This lies just above the brainstem and has long been suspected as the possible origin of headaches. It links the nervous system with the endocrine (hormone) system via the pituitary gland, resulting in the activation or suppression of organs such as the ovary, testes, and adrenal gland. It also controls basic functions such as hunger, thirst, and

body temperature. It is found in all vertebrates; in humans, it is about the size of an almond.

- **Pituitary gland:** This gland, which lies close to the hypothalamus, is even smaller: about the size of a pea. Its importance lies in the hormones that it secretes or controls. These include hormones for growth, sexual function, childbirth, lactation, thyroid function, fluid balance, and endorphins.

- **Pineal gland:** Sitting midline and not far from the hypothalamus, this tiny structure is even smaller than the preceding two — about the size of a rice grain. Known sometimes as 'the third eye', it is of interest in headaches for several reasons: it is connected to the trigeminal ganglia, it produces melatonin, and it is stimulated by darkness and suppressed by light. There is extensive literature on melatonin in medical conditions such as headache, autoimmune disorders, and seasonal affective disorder. The production of melatonin from the pineal gland may explain why many people seek darkness when they have a headache.

- **'Reticular formation':** This is old term for the structure in the brainstem that has to do with basic functions such as the sleep–wake cycle, and cardiac and vasomotor reflexes. It also filters incoming information. Its importance in the headache story is that it used to be regarded as having a role in the modulation of pain signals.

Nowadays, it is customary to refer to the various nuclei that together serve the functions once ascribed to the reticular formation. The word 'nucleus' refers to a kind of hub or junction point in the brainstem of neurons associated with one or more cranial nerves.

Some other components of the central nervous system are worth looking at in more detail, particularly the periaqueductal grey matter and the limbic system.

Periaqueductal grey matter (PAG)

The PAG is an area of the midbrain that surrounds the cerebral aqueduct (the structure within the brainstem that connects the third ventricle to the fourth). Although it is not large, it has several interesting functions, particularly in relation to headaches. These functions are, I think, relevant to my argument that headache is essentially a protective mechanism.

- **Defensive behaviour:** In rats, stimulation of certain parts of the PAG provokes a defensive response, whereas stimulation of other sites results in a passive, or 'tame', response.
- **Analgesia:** In experimental situations, if the PAG is stimulated, a chain of messenger molecules can be released, including 5-HT (serotonin) and enkephalins (also known as endorphins). This may inhibit the neuropeptide known as Substance P, thus blocking the pain signal from going higher up into the cerebral cortex. (Substance P is discussed further in Chapter 13.) Drugs such as heroin, morphine, pethidine, and oxycodone produce analgesia by acting at this site.
- **Reproductive behaviour:** Female reproduction is thought to be affected by the activation of PAG neurons.

- **Consciousness:** While the PAG is not the only means of consciousness, it seems to play an essential role in consciousness.

The limbic system

In common with the reticular formation, the concept of the limbic system represents a historic step in neuroscientists' attempts to understand the structure and function of the brain. Since 1878, when Paul Broca coined the term, it has been used to ascribe certain functions to an area of the brain that includes the hippocampus (involved in forming memories), the amygdala (involved in producing emotions), the anterior thalamic nuclei (involved in memory and learning), the septum pellucidum (a membrane separating the brain's right and left ventricles), and the olfactory and limbic cortex. Its functions are thought to include behaviours related to feeding, emotion, reproduction, and parenting. It is sometimes referred to as the 'paleomammalian complex' because it represents an advance on the 'reptilian brain', but is not as advanced as the 'neomammalian complex' (or neocortex), where language planning and perception take place.

Many neuroscientists challenge the notion of the limbic system and such models of brain function, regarding them as obsolete. The relevance of the limbic system to our discussion is that many have seen it as the link between mind and brain, or between psychiatry and neurology. Some think that an understanding of limbic physiology will explain how factors such as emotional trauma predispose us to headache and pain.

CRANIAL NERVES

As we have seen, the cranial nerves are part of the parasympathetic nervous system, carrying messages to and from the brain.

The trigeminal nerve

This nerve is a good starting point for relating anatomy to headache and facial pain. The trigeminal nerve is the fifth cranial nerve, and it is mainly a sensory nerve. Its job is to bring sensory information into the brain for processing. It has three main branches, from upper to lower:

- ophthalmic, serving the upper part of the face and the top of the head
- maxillary, serving the middle part of the face, including the upper jaw
- mandibular, serving the lower part of the face, including the lower jaw and the side of the head.

The trigeminal nerve carries information about the face, the eyes (including the conjunctiva and the cornea), the jaw, and the teeth. It also conveys messages from parts of the meninges (membranes) that cover the brain, the blood supply to the meninges, and parts of the scalp.

The three branches of the trigeminal nerve join up to form the trigeminal ganglion. From this ganglion, a single large root enters the brainstem. Nearby, a smaller root emerges that carries motor messages involved almost entirely with biting, chewing, and swallowing. (The one exception to this is a small branch to the middle ear.)

Sensory information is then carried downwards via the trigeminal nuclei, located within the brainstem, through to the upper end of the spinal cord, and back to the midbrain. (Although they primarily serve the trigeminal nerve, these trigeminal nuclei actually receive *all* the sensory information that is carried from the face, even when it travels in other cranial nerves such as the seventh, ninth, and tenth. This means that these nuclei have the complete sensory map of the face and mouth — touch, pain, position, and temperature.)

Further processing of this information occurs as the messages are passed higher up into the brain, to the cerebral cortex. Here, factors such as memory and emotional overlay add to the complexity of pain and headache.

If you consider how important it is to protect the face, teeth, eyes, and head, it becomes easy to understand why the trigeminal system is critical in understanding headaches.

The facial nerve

The facial nerve, the seventh cranial, is — as you would expect — primarily responsible for controlling facial muscles. We have seen that the trigeminal nerve largely controls the sensory messages from the face, but the facial nerve also carries some sensory information, such as that to do with taste and earlobe sensation.

The vestibulo-cochlear nerve

This is the eighth cranial nerve, and it carries information from the inner ear to the brain. It is a purely sensory nerve, and has two main functions: hearing and balance. The cochlear nerve (the acoustic nerve) is concerned with hearing, and the vestibular division is concerned with balance. Many people experience giddiness as part of their headaches. Ear infections, motion sickness, and adverse food reactions can all be associated with feelings of vertigo, recognised by many migraine sufferers as part of the lead-up to a headache.

The vagus nerve

The tenth cranial nerve was named 'vagus' from the Latin word for 'wandering'. With both motor and sensory fibres, it controls motion and sensations. It also has parasympathetic fibres that extend to almost all of the thoracic and abdominal organs. One of the main tasks of the vagus nerve is to communicate information about the state of the body's organs to the brain. This includes the heart, lungs, and gut.

The motor branches of the vagus nerve have a para-sympathetic action on heart rate, peristalsis (gut motility), and sweating. The neurotransmitter acetylcholine acts on a type of receptor called muscarinic to slow heart rate, open sphincters, aid digestion, and assimilate food.

For the relief of refractory migraine and cluster headaches, the implantation of electrodes that stimulate the vagus nerve has been trialled.[116] It is possible that acupuncture and acupressure work in a similar way.

In Chapter 5, we saw how mice with infectious colitis treated with the gut bacterium *Bifidobacterium longum* showed demonstrable stress reduction. The hypothesis was that neurotransmitters such as serotonin, which these bacteria help to produce, were able to 'talk' to the brain via the vagus nerve. This accords with the calming aspect of parasympathetic function, and fits in with the idea of the gut as the 'second brain'. You will remember that when the vagus nerve in the mice was cut, the beneficial effect of the bacteria was lost.

SPINAL NERVES

Spinal nerves are part of the peripheral nervous system, and are divided by area into cervical, thoracic, lumbar, and sacral. There are 31 pairs of spinal nerves, roughly corresponding to appropriate segments of the spinal column. Spinal nerves are mixed in function, carrying motor, sensory, and autonomic messages between the spinal cord and the rest of the body.

The motor functions supplied by any one spinal nerve are referred to as its 'myotome'. The sensory functions are expressed as its 'dermatome'. Abnormal sensation on the surface of the skin gives us information about which nerve may be involved. The allodynia (extreme sensitivity to touch; see Chapter 5) experienced by migraine sufferers is explained by activation of a related dermatome.

Spinal nerves relevant to headaches include the occipital nerve, particularly in relation to the types of headache known as occipital neuralgias. Recent research has also led to increased interest in the occipital nerves in relation to migraine.

WHERE IS THE PAIN COMING FROM?

To answer that question, we have to look at what is known as the trigemino-vascular system.

The trigemino-vascular system (TVS)

Collectively, the blood vessels associated with the trigeminal nerve, its ganglia, and the areas that its fibres pass through are referred to as the trigemino-vascular system. You may remember that the blood–brain barrier consists of cells on the surface of blood vessels that act like a membrane, separating the brain from the blood vessels that supply it. Events that take place in the TVS must pass through this barrier.

In terms of the neural pathways, some trigeminal fibres go straight up into the brain. Others take a much more indirect loop: down to the upper spinal cord and back up through the brainstem, midbrain, and finally the cortex.

When there is altered reactivity in these blood vessels, it starts a series of events that we will discuss in the next chapter, under the heading of cortical spreading depression. What brings about this changed state is the subject of much inquiry. We know that activation of the TVS releases chemicals known as neuromodulators, which cause dilation of the cerebral blood vessels. As these blood vessels dilate, the characteristic throbbing pain of the migraine begins. (This is the step that is targeted by the ergot alkaloid drugs, and underpins one of the actions of the triptans.)

In recent years, there has been a growing belief among researchers that the trigeminal nerve has a role to play in *all* kinds of primary headaches. It seems that in any kind of headache, the trigeminal nerve is likely to be flooding the brain with pain signals. For example, it has been claimed that dysfunction in the trigemino-vascular nociceptive (pain) regulation system is the cause of chronic daily headache.[117] What sets off the trigeminal nerve, and how it responds, may determine what kind of headache the person ends up with.[118]

The trigeminal nerve receives sensory information from the scalp, teeth, and face, and indirectly from the neck. Part of that information includes messages from the blood vessels of those regions. Information about pain is an obvious purpose of this system, but less obvious is the 'need' we have to know what is happening to our blood vessels. Perhaps they are part of a relay team that sends messages in the critical task of protecting the brain and the nervous system — indeed, the whole organism — from injury.

We might wonder why this pain pathway takes such a long journey, detouring via the spinal cord, the brainstem, and the midbrain. An obvious, if simplistic, reply is that it gives plenty of opportunity along the way for modification of the pain experience. After all, pain is useful if it sends a warning, but if it incapacitates you, it is anything but protective. When all is going well, this long journey does seem to have an important role in pain modification. This is where the PAG system, described in Chapter 10, which blocks the pain signal, becomes relevant. In 'normal' pain, there is a release of dampening agents that we know as endorphins. Just like the drug morphine, they work by binding to opioid receptor sites and blocking the release of Substance P. A similar effect is also achieved by the neurotransmitter GABA. (Both of these molecules are discussed further in Chapter 13.)

Glial cells

In Chapter 4, we were introduced to microglial cells as components of the blood–brain barrier. These cells are sometimes simply referred to as 'glial' cells. Microglia are one kind of glial cell.

Large nerves, such as the trigeminal, are surrounded by glial cells. These are 'housekeepers' in the health of brain cells; they repair damage when it occurs. If we look back at Diagram 1 in Chapter 2, in the lower left corner we see how both the release of glutamate and neuronal damage cause (micro)glial activation. So too does the consumption of opiates and foods with opiate properties. We have seen that vitamin B2 helps to prevent the release of glutamate; this and other supplements may support the glial cells while they undertake repair work on the brain cells. We know that in some cases chronic daily headache is the result of medication overuse, so we must be careful to avoid contributing to that problem. We can certainly avoid additives such as MSG.

When we discuss glial cells, and shortly, associated astrocytes, we are talking about cells found throughout the entire central nervous system. When they are on the surface of the blood vessels, they are contributing to the blood–brain barrier. Perhaps the 'barrier' in the TVS would be better seen as a forum for dialogue between the brain and anything arriving or leaving by its blood supply.

Glial cells need magnesium to maintain their normal potassium balance.[119] Loss or release of potassium is part of the cascade of events known as cortical spreading depression. As we have seen in Chapter 8, the modern diet is typically low in magnesium, and contains too much sodium and too little potassium. So headache sufferers have several options to help support their glial cells: watch their diet, take some B vitamins, lower their sodium input, and get some magnesium into them. They should certainly not be eating glutamate.

To know that your headaches may have caused low-grade brain damage would have once been a gloomy prospect. But in recent times, we have learned much about neuroplasticity — the brain's ability to regenerate neurons, which was once thought to be impossible. Earlier I recommended the book *The Brain that Changes Itself* by Norman Doidge. We know that the brain needs good nutrition and bodily exercise; we know that it can be affected by heavy metal toxicity and nutrient deficiencies. I think we should take a holistic and positive view to managing even the most intractable of chronic headaches.

The high prevalence of headache in our society provides fertile ground for the pharmaceutical industry to fund research and sell drugs. If you were stricken with recurrent cluster headaches, you might think it churlish of me to begrudge such research. Balance that against the fact that most headache sufferers prefer to avoid an excess of medication. Even where medication brings relief, they dislike feeling dependent on it, they dislike feeling 'drugged', and they dislike the side effects.

Where possible, it is my aim for my patients to free themselves from both drugs and headaches. I am not always successful, but sometimes it is easier than patients dared hope; we have already seen some of their stories.

We should be resolute in doing the safe and simple things.

I have said that glial cells are 'housekeepers', maintaining brain health, but they also have other functions. Here are some types of glial cells and their specialties.

- **Oligodendrocytes:** These are the chief maintenance workers for the insulation system around nerves — the myelin sheaths. Loss of myelination is the problem in disorders such as multiple sclerosis.
- **Microglia:** These are part of the immune system. They have been described as the 'resident macrophages' in the central nervous system. Macrophages are large white blood cells that are named from Greek words meaning 'big appetite', and in our bloodstream, they gobble up all manner of flotsam and jetsam. Microglia in the CNS can gobble up damaged cells, toxic chemicals, or infective invaders. They are also able to scan their territory and talk to the neurons that produce neurotransmitters such as serotonin and dopamine.
- **Astrocytes:** Although they do not have electrical activity, these are involved in the transmission of messages. Astrocyte dysfunction, leading to reduced clearing of glutamate, has been studied in the context of the progression of ALS, a form of motor-neuron disease.[120]

These glial cells are not only found in the central nervous system; they are widely distributed in the enteric nervous system, lending more evidence to the idea of the gut as our 'second brain'. Both microglia and astrocytes are known to release neuro-excitatory substances such as nitric oxide and inflammatory cytokines, and this makes them key players in headaches. The fact that glial cells have an immune function reminds us that the pain we experience may warn not only of a physical threat, but also of a chemical and/or an immunological threat.

The cardiovascular system

The most relevant aspects of this system have just been discussed under the heading 'The trigemino-vascular system'. However, there is a structural cardiac problem that warrants mention.

For some time now, it has been noted that people who have undergone surgery for a 'hole in the heart' have often lost their migrainous headaches. The most common cause of having a hole in the heart is the otherwise relatively benign condition known as patent foramen ovale (PFO). PFO is a developmental defect in that a hole, normally present in foetal development, fails to close off after birth — which it usually does as pressure in the heart and lungs changes once the infant is outside the mother's body. Indeed, a 2008 study, led by Doctor Stephanie Nahas and Doctor Stephen Silberstein at the Thomas Jefferson University Hospital in the United States, led to the startling claim that up to 66 per cent of chronic migraineurs had this condition.[121]

The most likely rationale for the headache would be that micro-emboli (tiny blood clots) were being generated by turbulent blood flow through the hole, triggering cortical spreading depression. Heart surgery to cure migraine seems a bit dramatic, but certainly, anyone with a (benign) heart murmur should consider assessment by a cardiologist interested in this area.

The musculoskeletal system

When we discuss stress as a trigger for migraine and a cornerstone of tension headache, its most obvious expression is through muscle contraction. Stress can be triggered by muscle pain, or can cause it.

There is an intriguing idea that muscles, bones, tendons, and ligaments can carry a 'memory' of pain through their nociceptive receptors. We will be discussing nociceptive receptors, which cause or react to pain, in the next chapter, but you will remember from Chapter 5, when we discussed complex regional pain syndrome, that it really is not possible, anatomically or biochemically, to separate pain, muscle tension, and stress from one another.

Dentition

Dental problems, teeth grinding, and jaw clenching may play a significant role in all forms of headache. Chapter 6 showed us that much of our health is dependent on the food we eat, and the diet for which we are 'designed' is very different from the diet that most Westerners consume. So it is not surprising that the temporo-mandibular joint, also known as the TMJ, may be the seat of many headaches. If we are raised on soft, processed foods, the growing jaw may not develop in accordance with nature's intention — which is for it to grind and masticate. The soft diet may not provide the nutritional building blocks for joint repair. It may lead to tooth decay and loss, as well as poor alignment of the jaw, and thus maldistribution and pressure on the TMJ.

As dysfunction of the joint develops, messages of pain and distress are relayed to the brain through the trigeminal nerve. The problem is exacerbated when a person, through stress or other causes, grinds their teeth or clenches their jaw during sleep — or even while awake. It is estimated that the average pressure on a tooth during normal eating is about 30 to 50 pounds per square inch (psi), but teeth grinding during sleep (bruxism) can produce a pressure up to 600 psi. This is why I think all headache sufferers would do well to visit a dentist to discuss whether any teeth or jaw problems may be contributing to their headaches.

The gastrointestinal system

The beginning of the gastrointestinal tract is of course the mouth, and I have just explained the importance of the jaw in headaches; thorough headache assessment should include a visit to a dentist, preferably one with an interest in head pain. The gut as an immune organ, producer of neurotransmitters, and a 'second brain' has been discussed earlier in this chapter. Gut bacteria play a key role in balancing our hormones, and therefore have relevance for hormonal headaches.

The role of gut bacteria was discussed in Chapter 5, when we saw how mice with infectious colitis treated with *Bifidobacterium longum* showed a reduction in stress.

The endocrine system

The endocrine system comprises the glands in our bodies that secrete hormones directly into the bloodstream. These glands include the pancreas, pituitary, thyroid, adrenals, and gonads. Less commonly thought of are the pineal gland, which is the primary source of melatonin, and the enteric paraganglia.

The latter is a bit of a mouthful, but it refers to the actions of the ganglia (nerve tissues that produce messenger molecules that enter the bloodstream rather than communicating through the neural network).

The relevance of endocrine glands for the headache story is apparent right from the sex hormones to the stress hormones and to the role of melatonin in headaches and sleep. They are discussed in Chapters 3 and 7.

CHAPTER 12
Headache Chemistry I: molecules and amines

'To think is to practise brain chemistry.'
DEEPAK CHOPRA

We start the chemistry story by looking at the pain pathways in migraine. As Chapters 1 and 10 have shown, the classification of headaches is not clear-cut, and an understanding of migraine seems to throw light on a range of headache types.

CORTICAL SPREADING DEPRESSION (CSD)

An episode of migraine consists of a series of biochemical events, referred to as the 'migraine cascade'. This process is not fully understood. The current thinking about it is best summarised thus: something initiates a chain of events in the brainstem, in the area that many still refer to as the reticular formation (see Chapter 11). This activates the trigemino-vascular system and leads to a chain reaction of biochemical events.

Whatever triggers the brainstem activity (the neuro-chemistry gets very complex here), the next step is a wave of electrical depolarisation that goes right across the cerebral cortex. Known as cortical spreading depression, this wave leads to a massive release of potassium and glutamate. The TRESK gene (discussed in Chapter 2) is thought to exert its effects by its action on this cascade.

CSD has been studied in experiments involving animals. It is initiated by such diverse events as blunt trauma to the head, exposure to excitatory amino acids or large amounts of potassium, or the release of a factor known as endothelin-1, derived from the lining of blood vessels. Recently, it has been suggested that tiny blood clots might trigger CSD. Spasms of blood vessels during an attack have been suspected of leading to clots, but the idea that the reverse is possible is interesting. People with certain polymorphisms of the MTHFR gene are more at risk of clotting, so this may possibly explain how this gene increases the risk of migraine and stroke. It might also explain why there is value in informing the brain of what is happening to our blood vessels.[122]

Recent research has made a connection between an increase in white matter lesions in the brain and a history of severe headache of any kind. Correlation seemed to be highest between stroke and the number of lesions. Patients with migraine with aura and patent foramen ovale (Chapter 11) appeared to be worst affected.[123] The study raises more questions than answers, but it is another step in our understanding of headache.

To summarise the headache process: something happens in the brainstem, possibly as the result of some incoming information via a nerve such as the trigeminal nerve. This may activate the TVS. The information gets sent to the conscious brain. As it passes through the midbrain and the periaquaductal grey matter (see Chapter 11), there is opportunity for the pain control system to swing into action. If the pain control system is not activated, a headache follows.

WHAT DO YOU MEAN WHEN YOU TALK ABOUT BRAIN CHEMISTRY, DOCTOR?

Shortly we will have a detailed look at the messenger molecules that the body uses to communicate from one part of itself to another. We first met these messenger molecules in Chapter 3, when we were looking at food links to headache. There we saw the overlaps between chemicals that our body makes (neurotransmitters, hormones, cytokines, and the like), chemicals that exist in nature, and synthetic chemicals. These chemicals have a lot of similarities, and may affect our experience of headache.

Chapter 13 focuses on the story of the messenger molecules relevant to human (and animal) chemistry. Before that detailed discussion, let us take an overview of the compounds we are talking about. Although we are separating them here for purposes of discussion, remember that there is a lot of overlap between the natural world, the human-made, and the human applications of this chemistry.

Throughout this book I have used the word 'molecule' as if it were part of everyday language, and for some, it will be.

But perhaps it is useful to provide a working definition of the term.

All matter is made up of atoms, such as hydrogen, oxygen, calcium, zinc, or magnesium. Each atom is like a tiny solar system, with a nucleus at the centre, and electrons orbiting around the nucleus. When one atom joins up to another, such as one oxygen to another oxygen (represented as O_2), or one oxygen joined to a nitrogen (NO), it is called a 'molecule'. Three atoms may join up to give us H_2O ... or water. Many atoms can also combine to give us a very large molecule, a 'macromolecule'. Insulin is an enormous molecule, made up of hundreds of atoms.

At the risk of turning this into a chemistry dissertation, the points to be made here are:

- molecules are the stuff of which matter is made, using atoms as the basic building blocks
- some molecules are produced in nature and some are only synthetic (for example, petroleum is natural, but after chemical processing, it can be turned into pesticides and cosmetics)
- both natural and synthetic molecules can impact on human health.

NATURE'S MOLECULES

Nature's molecules are everywhere — in plants, in the natural environment, and in animals, including humans.

Biologically active amines

We begin our survey of nature's chemicals by looking at amines. Amines are small molecules, and they join with other simple molecules to make amino acids — the building blocks of proteins.

Many foods, especially those that are fermented or aged, contain amines. Chapter 6 gives a comprehensive list of amine-rich foods. Amino acids are the basic chemical of many of our neurotransmitters, and the interaction between dietary amines, on the one hand, and our neurotransmitters, on the other, is central to the headache story. The relevant neurotransmitters will be discussed shortly. We will see that many, such as dopamine, end with the word 'amine'.

Caffeine

Caffeine is one of the best-known amines — especially in the context of headache. It belongs in a class of compounds known as methylxanthines. Other methylxanthines include paraxanthine, theobromine, and theophylline. They are found in coffee, tea, chocolate, energy drinks, cola, yerba mate, and guarana. In plants, methylxanthines act as a pesticide, and you will find that coffee grounds are an effective way of keeping slugs and snails off the garden.

Methylxanthines have been linked to headaches of all kinds, as well as to breast pain, benign breast disease, restless legs, nausea, vomiting, panic disorder, and heart rhythm disturbances.

Caffeine is highly addictive. Caffeine withdrawal often proves a stumbling block in an elimination diet. Patients can go cold turkey on suspect foods, but to do so with caffeine can court disaster; the caffeine-withdrawal headache is enough to stop them at the outset.

Dopamine

Dopamine is well known as a neurotransmitter affecting mood. Several foods help our bodies to make dopamine, and they are sometimes described as 'dopaminergic'. (For a list of foods containing dopamine, see Chapter 6.) These are all healthy foods, and I am not suggesting that we should avoid them; the point is that when someone identifies a food link to their headaches, doctors should take it seriously and look for patterns.

Histamine

We saw in Chapter 9 that some headaches are described as 'histamine headaches', and in these cases a low-histamine diet may be prescribed. We will discuss histamine later in this chapter, so the point here is simply that the molecule exists out there in the natural world.

Food sources of histamine include fermented food, fresh tuna, and gouda cheese. For a more comprehensive list of foods containing histamine, see Chapter 6.

Nitrosamine

Nitrates and nitrites will be discussed shortly, when we look more closely at food additives. However, nitrates also occur naturally in meat and vegetables, and can be converted to nitrites by bacteria in our mouths. These combine with certain amines from our foods in the acidic environment of the stomach to produce nitrosamine.

Nitrosamine, as the name implies, is an amine. It is also reputed to be a carcinogen. Tobacco contains nitrosamine, and it is one of the major types of carcinogens in tobacco. Smoking is a well-known risk factor for headache.

The addition of nitrites to cured meats greatly increases the formation of nitrosamines, and bacon and hot dogs regularly appear in lists of foods linked to headaches. (See the section on 'hot-dog headache' in Chapter 4.)

Phenylethylamine

This is a biological amine that can raise blood pressure. The alkaloid salsolinol, which appears in cocoa and chocolate, is a derivative of phenylethylamine. It is avoided as part of the low-amine diet in some protocols for headache management.

Serotonin

We will discuss serotonin in some detail in the next chapter, when we look at molecules relevant to human/animal chemistry. Naturally occurring serotonin is found in various foods, which have been removed from some successful elimination diets. For a list of foods containing serotonin, see Chapter 6.

Tryptamine

Tryptamine is another biogically active amine found in foods such as cheese and tomatoes, and in various other fruits and vegetables. Tryptamine does not appear to be as reactive as tyramine when consumed in large doses.

Tyramine

Tyramine occurs widely in plants and animals. Humans can make tyramine from the amino acid tyrosine in foods, or ingest it in foods that contain high levels of it (it is often produced during fermentation or decay). Foods containing considerable amounts of tyramine include those that are spoiled, pickled, aged, smoked, yeasty, or fermented. (A more comprehensive list of such foods is in Chapter 6.) The point is that these characterise a modern diet, whereas the diet of our hunter-gatherer ancestors was low in tyramine.

The effects of a high tyramine load include the constriction of blood vessels, leading to elevation of blood pressure and rapid heart rate. Tyramine acts by releasing related neurotransmitters, dopamine, nor-adrenalin, and adrenalin. It is also possible that it may act directly as a neurotransmitter in its own right. A 2007 research review showed that both migraine and cluster headaches were characterised by an increase in circulating neurotransmitters or neuromodulators, such as tyramine, in the hypothalamus, amygdala, and dopaminergic system during an attack.[124]

Tyramine is broken down in the body by the enzyme monoamine oxidase (MAO; see Chapter 10). Since the 1950s, MAO inhibitors (MAOIs) have been used for the treatment of depression, anxiety, and panic disorders. If people on these medications eat cheese, they can experience a 'cheese headache'. High doses of tyramine in foods such as ripe cheese, when coupled with MAOIs that block the breakdown of the tyramine, can lead to hypertensive crisis — a severe increase in blood pressure that can lead to a stroke. (This is comparable to the 'serotonergic syndrome' discussed in Chapter 13 under 'Serotonin'; see also Chapter 9.) This happens when tyramine triggers the release of adrenalin, nor-adrenalin, and dopamine. People who are not taking MAOIs sometimes report that their headaches are helped by a low-tyramine diet.

Phenolic compounds

Most foods have phenolic compounds in them. The structure of a phenol is shown in Diagram 5. They are weakly acidic compounds with a particular arrangement of hydrogen and carbon atoms. (Carbolic acid, used as an antiseptic and disinfectant, and known as phenol, is one of them.) Some of the amines we have just looked at are phenolic structures.

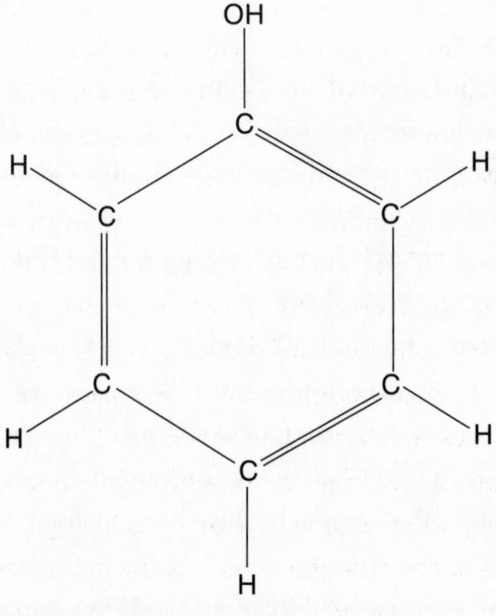

Diagram 5: the structure of a phenol

Mother Nature makes use of phenolic compounds in many ways. Dietary phenols are significant antioxidants, and in plants they are there to protect against the sun's radiation and other sources of oxidative stress. But they protect us too. They are instrumental in fighting cancers and other diseases related to ageing. Polyphenolic compounds such as flavones, isoflavones, bioflavonoids, tannins, catechins, and anthocyanins are the subject of much current research in this regard.

Dietary phenols are found in high concentration in tea, red fruits, grapes, tomatoes, and cocoa. (For a more comprehensive list of foods high in phenols, see Chapter 6.) The antioxidant potential of these foods is considerable. The flipside for some people is the risk of headaches — and also phenol sensitivity, which will be discussed shortly.

Alkaloids

Salsolinol, mentioned on page 275 under the heading 'Phenylethylamine', is an alkaloid in cocoa and chocolate. We also met some other members of the alkaloid group when we discussed caffeine and chocolate: methylxanthines. Both salsolinol and methylxanthines are part of the large family of naturally occurring alkaloids.

Medical use of natural alkaloids goes back a long way, and use of synthetic alkaloids has followed more recently. Morphine, caffeine, ergotamine, and nicotine are all alkaloids. Their effects are many and various. We use them as drugs for established headache, but they can also be the cause of headaches.

We were introduced to ergot alkaloids in Chapter 1, with the drug ergotamine. The medicinal history of alkaloids began with ergot, which was derived from a group of fungi that grows on rye and other grains. The alkaloids produced by the fungus can cause the condition of 'ergotism', seen in humans and animals that consume infected grains. Because in medieval times the monks at St Anthony's Hospital in France specialised in treating ergotism victims with plant extracts, ergotism is sometimes known by the name 'St Anthony's Fire'. The toxicity of some mushrooms is due to the alkaloids in them.

The alkaloid group encompasses the *Solanaceae* family. This family includes toxic plants such as deadly nightshade, and food plants such as potato, eggplant, tomato, and capsicum. Tobacco also belongs to this family. Nightshade sensitivity has been linked to arthritis and migraine. So if someone is getting headaches after eating foods from the *Solanaceae* family, we need to ask whether the reaction is through the immune system via IgG (see Chapter 3), or whether it is a response to the alkaloid content of the food, or some other factor again.

Many other foods implicated in the causation of migraine and tension headaches also have alkaloid and opiate properties. These include gluten (gluteomorphin), casein from milk (caseomorphin), and eggs. Foods such as citrus and tomato are said to have alkaloid properties, and may cause mischief, as they activate opiate receptors on glial cells (see Chapter 11).[125]

Salicylates

Salicylates were discussed in Chapter 3. They are aspirin-like molecules that occur widely in foods, and are produced, as we have seen, as part of the plant's immune system. Some of the tastiest foods are those that are naturally high in salicylates. Our ancestors probably had salicylates in small doses, but not so in our modern diet. To compound the problem, many food colourings and additives have salicylate chemistry.

It is perhaps easier to list foods that are *low* in salicylates than to do the reverse. Cereals, meat, fish, and dairy products have no significant levels; nor do peas, chickpeas, dried beans, lentils, potatoes, and swedes. By contrast, spices are often high in salicylates. For a more comprehensive list of foods high in salicylates, see Chapter 6.

Children with allergies, hyperkinetic children, adults with irritable bowel syndrome, and people with headaches are often put on a low-salicylate diet. The effects range from minimal through to almost complete resolution of the problem. Sometimes a low-amine diet is followed at the same time. This leaves individuals a very narrow choice because the two food groups can be quite different — when both salicylates and amines are removed, not much is left. *Friendly Food*, an excellent book produced by the allergy clinic at Royal Prince Alfred Hospital in Sydney, is helpful in this regard (further publication details are in the further reading list near the end of this book).

When we look at the lists of foods high in salicylates, we notice that many hunter–gatherer foods appear. Surely these foods constitute the most 'natural' diet of all? But perhaps the problem is that we don't eat these foods in their proper season. Is our food picked green, or is there something wrong with our gut?

Aspirin is also a salicylate, and some of us are sensitive to it. This may be genetic, but it is possible that the effect of commercial aspirin increases gut permeability and makes us sensitive to it and a whole range of otherwise innocuous food substances.

SYNTHETIC MOLECULES

With the increased industrial production of food and an ever-growing understanding of chemistry, it has become customary to add a variety of synthetic molecules to food. Some of these have a valuable purpose, such as food preservation, and some are there to help sales by boosting taste. All of them have potential for negative health effects.

Artificial colours

In 2007, the UK medical journal *The Lancet* published the results of a study led by Professor Jim Stevenson from the University of Southampton.[126] The researchers were investigating the following food additives to look at the effects they might have on hyperactivity in children:

- allura red AC (E129) (FD&C Red #40): an orange-red food dye
- carmoisine (E122): a red colouring, often used in jellies
- ponceau 4R (E124): a red colouring
- sunset yellow (E110) (FD&C Yellow #6): colouring, often found in squash drinks
- sodium benzoate (E211): preservative
- tartrazine (E102) (FD&C Yellow #5): yellow colouring
- quinoline yellow (E104): yellow colouring [127]

For many years, people have followed the Feingold Diet, which excludes — among other things — artificial colours and additives such as those in this list. The conditions treated include asthma, skin disorders, hyperkinetic behaviour, and headaches. For just as many years, various medical cynics, not to mention the food industry, have been at pains to 'prove' the Feingold Diet invalid, despite some excellent studies with impressive results.[128] Politicians, always loath to stand up to big industry, have been unwilling to legislate against these additives.

But it seems that attitudes in Europe are at last turning, and Stevenson's study has helped bring this about. In April 2008, the UK's Food Standards Agency called for a voluntary removal of the artificial colours (but not the preservative sodium benzoate) by 2009. Furthermore, it recommended that they should be phased out in food and drink in the European Union. By 2010, the six listed colours were still legal under EU legislation, but in the United Kingdom they had to carry additional warnings.

Jim Stevenson is said to have commented that these additives should be regarded as being as harmful to the developing brain as lead![129] Some people point out that there are children who consume a lot of food additives and seem to be unaffected. My reply is that not all children are slow hydroxylators, poor acetylators, or have other vulnerable detox enzymes.

Tartrazine (E102)

As a doctor, I have seen many children come into the emergency room on a Saturday afternoon after going to a birthday party. Their symptoms include acute asthma, abdominal pain, and rash. It is not hard to make the link to tartrazine when you ask about yellow-coloured party food.

At a personal level, I have experienced several classic migraine attacks after eating food that had unsuspected E102 in it. The brightly coloured sweets and soft drinks are easy to identify, but I have been caught out by custard powder, cheese, salad dressing, and — unbelievably — clear-coloured soda water.

The green colouring that affected my patient Marjorie, in Chapter 1, appears to have been a combination of blue food colouring and tartrazine.

Some of my headache patients have made the connection between this additive and their experience of headache. Others seem genuinely surprised that such a thing would be possible. Often the response is, 'Why is it allowed?' Why indeed.

Interestingly, tartrazine cross-reacts with aspirin, so people who know that they are aspirin-sensitive should avoid this food colour.[130] Chemically speaking, it is an azo dye, a derivative of aromatic sulphonic acid. I do not know whether the intolerance is connected to sulphur sensitivity (discussed later in this chapter), but the chemical link between aspirin and tartrazine is well recognised.

A 2010 *Sydney Morning Herald* article stated: 'A report this year by the US Centre for Science in the Public Interest, titled *Food Dyes: a rainbow of risks*, found that colourings can pose a risk of cancer, hyperactivity in children, and allergies, and called for them to be banned across America.'[131] To these problems, I would add headache. Overstimulation of the nervous system is at the heart of hyperactivity, and also, as we have seen, of many headache events. These colours are non-foods, and have proved themselves so harmful that I believe they have no place at all in human diets.

Erythrosine (E127)

When I first met Doctor Robert Buist, a few things stuck in my mind and have never left. One was his explanation of the chemistry surrounding E102; another, his explanation of the chemistry of erythrosine.

Buist's 1986 book, *Food Chemical Sensitivity*, cites studies that suggest that E127 inhibits the uptake of dopamine, choline, GABA, glycine, glutamate, and nor-adrenalin. These neurotransmitters perform various actions, which are discussed elsewhere in this book. The point here is that we are looking at a chemical that can interefere with the balance of our neurotransmitters.

Furthermore, this compound, a xanthene derivative with four iodine atoms stuck on it, has a structural resemblance to thyroxine (which also bears four iodine atoms). Erythrosine was shown to have a dose-related thyroxine effect in animal studies.[132] This means that the animals behaved as if they were thyrotoxic: they were agitated and irritable, with a fast heart rate.

I could not believe that we were giving food colours to kids that could make them act as if they were on thyroid hormones. The powers that be eventually came to this realisation as well, and a phasing-out process began in 1991. Glacé (cocktail) cherries were the notable exception, and were still allowed.

This strike for sanity is important, as a 2011 review on erythrosine safety also acknowledged that it affects thyroid function and causes tumours in the thyroid gland of rats.[133] Yet it is a concern that the guidelines still allow cocktail cherries, which they state should not exceed a consumption of 0.1 milligrams per kilogram of body weight per day. This level equals about 30 cocktail cherries. I do not find the authorities' comment, 'which is unlikely to occur on a frequent basis', in any way reassuring. What if you like cocktail cherries? What if kids think of them as lollies? What about your inherited detox enzymes?

Allura red (E129)

E129 is another azo dye, but it lacks the iodine atoms of erythrosine. It is one of the colours studied in the *Lancet* review.

As of 2014, E129 is still widely available in Australia. Amazingly, not all that long ago it was in a popular children's breakfast cereal. I remember a 1990s ABC television documentary on attention-deficit disorder, in which recalcitrant children just about swung from the chandeliers as the earnest presenters (a psychiatrist, and a paediatrician and journalist) explained why these children could not be calmed down without Ritalin. The cameras caught, but did not focus on, the cereal packet on the table and the children's breakfast bowls. At that time, this particular cereal also contained E100, E110, and E133. Today's version of this cereal has replaced them with more natural and safer colours. However, the colours can still be found in the confectionery section of the supermarket.

Artificial preservatives

Once upon a time, sugar and salt were the main preservatives used in food. Large doses of these are not good for the body, but the food industry has come up with many alternatives that carry their own health problems. We will look at the most notable.

Benzoic acid derivatives (E210–13)

Benzoic acid compounds occur naturally in foods such as berries, plums, cinnamon, and cloves. As synthetic additives, they are found in a range of acidic foods, including carbonated drinks, fruit juices, and prepared salads. They are used because they help to control yeasts, moulds, and some bacteria. The link to headaches is well recognised.

Nitrates and nitrites (E249–50)

As we have seen earlier in this chapter, nitrates and nitrites exist in nature, like benzoic acid derivatives. Nitrates occur naturally in foods like red meat, and to a lesser extent in vegetables. But with the use of synthetic fertilisers in agribusiness, there has been a rise in the levels of nitrates throughout the food chain in recent decades. We are seeing higher levels in foods such as leafy greens, beetroot, celery, and radish. They are also added during food processing, especially to cured meats.

Nitrates may be converted to nitrites when food spoils, by bacteria in our mouths, or by intestinal bacteria after consumption. The problem comes when nitrates or nitrites interact in the gut with amines to produce nitrosamines. Nitrosamines are rated as highly carcinogenic, especially in terms of the link to gastrointestinal cancers. This risk may be reduced by the antioxidant effects of vitamins A, C, and E in the form of fresh yellow and green vegetables. We have to balance the cancer risks against the risk of food poisoning if we did not use preservatives in processed foods and meats.

Nitrites not only increase the formation of nitrosamines; they also cause blood vessels to dilate. Bacon and hot dogs, both high in nitrites, regularly appear in lists of foods linked to headaches. (See 'hot dogs', Chapter 4.)

Sulphur derivatives (E220–28)

Sometimes patients say that they are allergic to sulphur. This is not strictly correct, and we can end up in a chemistry debate. Let's get some clarification.

First, the spelling: American English spells the word with an 'f' (*sulfur* and so on) but British and Australian English usage is 'ph' (*sulphur* and so on). I follow the Australian convention, but the products you buy, and the medical literature, will vary in spelling according to the country of origin.

The compounds of concern include sulphur dioxide, sodium sulphite, sodium bisulphite, potassium bisulphite, sodium metabisulphite, and potassium metabisulphite. At the right acidity level (pH), these derivatives will release sulphur dioxide.

- **Sulphur**, in its atomic form, is essential to life. Plants need it for growth and function, and so do we. It is present in the sulphur-containing amino acids: cysteine, taurine, and methionine. Atomic sulphur is not relevant to any discussion on allergy or sensitivity.

- **Sulphonamide** antibiotics gave rise to the term 'sulphur allergy' to describe a true allergic response. While these antibiotics are no longer in common use, some other drugs have sulphonamide structures within them and can cause a cross-reactive allergic response. Drugs in this category (along with some brand names that you might know them by) include sulfasalazine, thiazide diuretics, frusemide (Lasix), sulfonylurea (Tolbutamide), anti-diabetic agents, sumatriptan (Imigran), and celecoxib (Celebrex).
- **Sulphites**, in the form of sulphur dioxide and metabisulphite, are used as preservatives in food, wine, and packaged salad leaves. Sulphites can cause hypersensitivity and intolerance reactions. Sulphites occur naturally, but rarely in the doses seen in food additives.
- **Sulphates**, such as magnesium sulphate (Epsom salts) and morphine sulphate, do not cause problems to people with sulphonamide or sulphite allergy or sensitivity.

Our bodies need sulphur. However, sulphur in the form of metabisulphite preservatives may be toxic not only to bacteria and moulds, but also to some of us. Migraine patients, and probably asthmatics, should avoid sulphur derivatives.

With all of this in mind, we need to look at how sulphur works in our bodies. To understand this, you may want to first go back to Chapter 10, which explains toxicity and bio-transformation. We saw there that the body uses enzymes to detoxify problematic compounds, and that these enzymes are classified as either phase-1 or phase-2.

Detoxifying sulphur compounds

Sulphur compounds may be sprayed onto your food, put in as legal additives, be used to dry fruits and vegetables, or be loaded into wines and soft drinks. They may end up lining cans for fish or the plastic bags that will hold fresh fish. They may be in the ice that the fish sits on in the market. The solution is to buy fish and vegetables fresh, not canned, and wash them well before cooking and consumption.

If you are unlucky enough to live near a power plant, either coal- or oil-fired, you may be inhaling sulphur dioxide on a regular basis. Even your doctor may be pressing sulphur on you: the drugs we use to treat the illnesses caused by sulphites — migraine, irritable bowel syndrome, asthma, and behavioural disturbances in children — may themselves contain sulphites.

When your body encounters problematic sulphur compounds, whether the source of the compound is natural or synthetic, the protective enzymes go to work. Let us look at two of them.

- **Phase 1 — sulphite oxidase:** Also known as SUOX, this enzyme turns the more toxic sulphites into non-toxic sulphates, thus allowing the body to excrete surplus sulphur. Variations in the gene that produces this enzyme are suspected to make some people more vulnerable to the toxic effects of sulphur drugs, sulphite additives, and sulphur-containing gases.

The enzyme needs molybdenum to work properly. Taking supplements of the mineral molybdenum (which is low in the typical Australian diet) may help.

• **Phase 2 — sulphotransferases:** A transferase, as the name implies, is an enzyme that transfers a chemical from one substance to another. The sulphotransferases belong to the phase-2 enzyme group, and one of them has the jaw-breaking name phenolsulphotransferase. It takes available sulphur and attaches (transfers) it to a toxic substance as a means of getting rid of the toxic waste.

Sulphation, or 'sulphonation', is not just a way of getting rid of poisons, but also of building structural proteins and glycoproteins. The compounds that are metabolised like this include: phenolic compounds in the diet; catecholamines (neurotransmitters); some steroid molecules, such as oestrogen; environmental poisons; and medications. It has been estimated that up to 20 per cent of the population are genetically 'slow sulphonaters'. They tend to be more chemically sensitive and more hormone sensitive, and to have more adverse food reactions.

Detoxifying phenols and amines

Both phenols and (dietary) amines require this same phase-2 process of conjugation. They too are sulphonated with phenolsulphotransferase. The gene for making this enzyme is polymorphic. Let us look at it now more closely, because we have seen in earlier chapters that people with headache may be prescribed a low-chemical diet, and this may mean the exclusion of (phenolic) amines.

Unless phenolsulphotransferase is working at its best, various phenolic amines can cause us trouble. Some of us have difficulty metabolising amines because we have been born with a less efficient version of this gene. Such individuals also have trouble metabolising foods high in phenols.

Markers for phenol intolerance include headache, odd rashes, red ears, and, in children, inappropriate behaviour and laughter, and night-time waking. Phenol problems are sometimes seen in children with autism. Doctors treating phenol-sensitive autistic children hear reports of them giggling in their bedrooms in the middle of the night for no obvious reason. Children with allergies often have dark rings around the eyes, possibly because they lack this enzyme, which is required to break down the products of haemoglobin, such as the pigment bilirubin. The enzyme deficiency contributes to the dark rings, and helps us to identify that certain foods are causing the allergic reactions.

But even if we have the more efficient version of phenolsulphotransferase, something else can go wrong. A report in the *British Journal of Pharmacology* indicated that an extract of six different types of red wine contained a substance that strongly inhibited phenolsulphotransferase.[134] Other foods that inhibit this enzyme include oranges, grapefruit, spinach, radish, beetroot, pumpkin, peppers, bananas, cheese, chocolate, and tomatoes. Salicylates, and food dyes with salicylate structures, also act as inhibitors. Even vitamin B6 and molybdenum in excess can do the same things, so again we see the importance of balance among different elements.

By contrast, magnesium supports phenolsulpho-transferase, and this is one of many ways in which magnesium might act to raise the headache threshold.

It is possible that phenolsulphotransferase becomes more efficient in the presence of additional sulphate ions. If this is the case, it shows yet again how our 'weaker' genes can be supported by a healthy diet. People with a deficiency of sulphate may be helped by sulphur-containing amino acids such as cysteine (found in egg yolks, red peppers, garlic, onion, broccoli, and brussels sprouts) and taurine (found in shellfish, eggs, and meat). Autistic children often react badly to opioid foods such as casein and gluten, but taurine has been observed to have an anti-opioid and calming effect on them.

Baths containing magnesium sulphate (Epsom salts) have helped calm agitated autistic children. Both the magnesium and the sulphate ions are thought to be involved. It is interesting to note that some studies on the effect of magnesium in migraine used oral magnesium sulphate. While the magnesium is considered the biologically active element, perhaps the sulphate component was lending support to the activity of this enzyme.

Flavour enhancers

You would be forgiven for thinking that the flavours of fresh, natural, healthy food did not need 'enhancing'. The food that kept our forebears alive was rendered tastier by, at most, the use of salt, sugar, and spices. But now other chemicals can be added. The most common of these are molecules based on glutamate. And here we run into the fuzzy borders between 'natural' and 'synthetic', and 'good' and 'bad', chemicals.

E621, MSG, and glutamate

Many people find that they get sick whenever they eat in a restaurant, and one cause of this might be monosodium glutamate (MSG). If you add a sodium atom to a molecule of glutamate, you have monosodium glutamate.

We met glutamate in the early chapters of this book. Glutamate, it should be understood, can be derived from the amino acids glutamine and glutamic acid, and it was introduced in Chapter 2 in connection with the gene EAAT2. So it is *not* a synthetic product, although it can be synthesised or made in a laboratory.

These amino acids serve important functions in the human body, which we will discuss shortly. First, we need to look at how glutamate came to such prominence in the modern diet.

Glutamic acid was first identified in 1866 by a German chemist, Karl Ritthausen. In 1907, it was isolated by a Japanese researcher at Tokyo University, Kikunae Ikeda, from *kombu*, a form of seaweed used as stock in many traditional Japanese dishes. He identified it as the source of the fifth taste, after salt, sweet, bitter, and sour. Referring to it as 'umami', he developed a method of mass production, which he patented.

The effect of glutamate can be described as 'moreish', and savoury foods that are naturally high in glutamate — peanuts, seaweed, cheese, and tomato concentrate — certainly have this quality. The manufacturers of snack foods were quick to add it to their products, and nowadays it can be difficult to find snacks that are *free* from MSG in one form or another.

Too much glutamate

If glutamate is found widely in nature, what is the difficulty? Glutamate often comes bound to other amino acids, where it causes little problem. The issue seems to be with free glutamate. Both modern food-processing methods and the deliberate addition of free glutamate as a flavour enhancer may be turning a safe, natural chemical into one that is toxic to some individuals.

You might think that food-labelling laws would protect us, but the food industry has a vested interest in us finding their products moreish. As many people are now suspicious of MSG, the manufacturers avoid putting 'MSG' on the label, calling it 'hydrolysed protein'. Peanuts are a cheap and convenient protein source, and as free glutamate is released when they are hydrolysed commercially, they are often used to produce free glutamate that can escape being labelled as MSG. Too bad if you are sensitive to glutamate or allergic to peanuts.

Exactly how does glutamate give us a headache? It has been identified as one of the key molecules released during a migraine. The beginning of this chapter described the process known as cortical spreading depression, which culminates in the headache experience. You will remember that it is the release of potassium and excitatory glutamate that triggers the headache. In our gun-and-bullet analogy, it is this release that fires the headache gun.

We read in Chapter 2 that the EAAT2 gene is one of those most likely to be associated with common migraine. Its job is to *clear* glutamate from nerve synapses. The use of botox for migraine and other headaches is based on its ability to block the release of glutamate.

Balancing glutamate

Let's look more closely at glutamate. It can help us to get rid of surplus nitrogen, and it acts as an important excitatory neurotransmitter. Take a look at Diagram 6, below. Glutamate, as we have seen, can be present in the diet, and our bodies can make it from a biological compound known as alpha-ketoglutarate, one of the intermediates of the energy-producing cycle, which is shown in Diagram 1 on page 50.

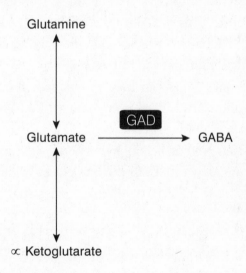

Diagram 6: glutamate

Normally, there is a nice balance between glutamate, glutamine, alpha-ketoglutarate, and another neurotransmitter — gamma-aminobutyric acid (GABA) — as each of these is able to convert into the others. In contrast to glutamine, which is an excitatory neurotransmitter, GABA is the body's 'calming' agent; it has been described as 'nature's Valium'.

It might also be noted that some neuroscientists have studied links between disturbance in glutamate metabolism, depression and suicidality. As this is beyond the scope of this book, all I can add here is a reinforcement of previous comments about links between mood and headache. However, enzymes carry out the interchange between these four products, and there are two important considerations here. First, these enzymes are produced by genes that have various polymorphisms — that is to say, more and less efficient forms. This includes the GAD genes, which were discussed in Chapter 10. Second, these enzymes can be inhibited by aluminium and by mercury.

Various substances can help to balance glutamate and GABA. Vitamin B12, grape seed extracts, Pycnogenol, and the amino acid taurine are all useful.[135] Do we wonder that vitamin B12 is proving helpful in migraine patients? But how do we become low in B12 in the first place? It may be poor diet, or we may have just inherited genes that need lots of B12.

We have already seen that taurine, found in shellfish and fresh fish, is sometimes given to autistic kids. This is why. It can calm them down when they are agitated because it helps them makes GABA, nature's Valium, rather than excitatory glutamate. Commercial preparations of GABA also exist.

So now we have this possible scenario: we may have inherited vulnerable enzymes in the first place; we are exposed to levels of metals unprecedented in human history; we have a diet low in fresh fish; and finally, we have an added load of glutamate dumped into our diet by a fast-food industry hungry for sales! The outcome is a surplus of neuronal excitement in the brain. This leads to increased sensitivity to sensory stimuli, such as light, sound, and pain, and to a loss of the calming GABA. Throw into this mix some E102 and other colours in snack foods, and what a surprise: we get a headache.

Is this bad design, bad genes — or bad diet?

So perhaps Deepak Chopra's words could be extended to, 'To eat is to possibly alter brain chemistry, even to the point of headache.'

CHAPTER 13
Headache Chemistry II: neurotransmitters and receptors

*'Nothing can be more incorrect than the assumption
one sometimes meets with, that physics has one method,
chemistry another, and biology a third.'*
THOMAS HUXLEY

Most of the molecules that are important in headache act as,
or are influenced by, neurotransmitters. Our bodies may make
these neurotransmitters. In addition, dietary ingredients or
environmental chemicals can mimic neurotransmitters, or
affect their function.

SMALL-MOLECULE NEUROTRANSMITTERS

The first group of neurotransmitters we will look at are small
molecules. These can be grouped into two: amino acids and
biogenic amines.

The amino acids include:

- glutamate (has an excitatory effect)
- gamma-aminobutyric acid, GABA (has an inhibitory, calming effect)
- glycine (has an inhibitory effect)
- aspartate (has an excitatory effect).

The biogenic amines include:

- dopamine (has an excitatory effect)
- nor-adrenalin (an excitatory monoamine)
- adrenalin (has an excitatory effect)
- histamine (has an excitatory effect)
- serotonin (an excitatory monoamine).

From this list, dopamine, nor-adrenalin, and adrenalin (also referred to as nor-epinephrine and epinephrine) are collectively referred to as 'catecholamines'. Stimulant drugs are often catecholamine analogues. Let us look at some of these neurotransmitters in more detail.

Glutamate and GABA

The first two neurotransmitters in the amino-acids list were discussed under 'Flavour enhancers' in Chapter 12. I include them here only for completion, and to remind the reader that while the temptation in the headache debate may be to see them as 'the bad guy' and 'the good guy' respectively, this is not necessarily the case. The issue is the balance between them.

Dopamine

This neurotransmitter is connected with a feeling of focus and wellbeing. We can make it in our bodies from the dietary amino-acid precursors phenylalanine and tyrosine. Such conversion reactions depend on the presence of nutrients such as folic acid, niacin, iron, and vitamin B6.

Dopamine is thought to play a role in various headaches. A 2006 study investigated the role of dopamine chemistry in some headaches, and the authors concluded: 'Our results support the hypothesis that the dopaminergic system is impaired in migraine and cluster headache', suggesting that high blood levels of dopamine may represent an abnormal biochemical trait of these headaches.[136]

As with all neurotransmitters, the key is balance. Too little dopamine and we feel anxious. Too much is associated with a whole spectrum of other medical disorders, including headache. Two drugs used in treating migraine, prochlorperazine and metoclopramide, act as dopamine antagonists. Many substances function by stimulating dopamine receptor sites, or mimicking the action of dopamine. Chocolate, nicotine, and alcohol are examples. We like the feel-good effect of these drug-foods, but headache may be the price we pay. Alcohol and cigarettes are also well-known associates of migraine and cluster headache.

In Chapter 12, we saw that chocolate contains an alkaloid called salsolinol, a psychoactive compound that might be included in chocolate addiction.[137] Although many migraine and cluster headache sufferers can get away with eating modest amounts of chocolate, I have found that most are affected to some extent. Over time, various researchers who have set out to see if chocolate is a provoker of migraine have found it wanting. There is a methodological problem here: to disguise the chocolate, it has often been administered in capsule form. This would be an appropriate test method if it were an IgE reaction of the immune system (discussed in Chapter 3). However, if the immune reaction has an IgG basis, it may be delayed, or it may show a monotonic dose response curve. That is to say, you have to eat enough of the stuff and wait long enough for the headache to appear. And if the reaction is outside the immune system altogether — if it is dopamine-related — then the response may be unpredictable because it will depend on the interaction with other neurotransmitters that happen to be around at any one point in time.

Histamine

Histamine is one of the biologically active amines that can be found in our food or produced in our bodies. We have seen some headaches described as 'histamine headaches', so what is it that histamine does in the body?

Histamine acts on receptors in the lungs to cause bronchoconstriction (airway spasm) and it does this by stimulating the smooth muscles of the airways to contract. Histamine is also a powerful capillary dilator, giving rise to facial flushing and urticarial rashes (hives). We know that blood pressure can sometimes drop dramatically as part of a histamine response. In relation to headaches, we should also note that histamine can cause a rise in pressure within the cerebrospinal fluid. When histamine is injected, nausea, vomiting, stomach pains, and intense headaches occur.

The body makes histamine from the precursor amino acid histidine, and sometimes we eat foods high in histamine and histidine. Although our bodies can make histamine from histidine, Mother Nature has her control systems: the conversion of histidine to histamine is inhibited by iodine.[138] Could the rise in the numbers of children who seem to be allergic to everything have anything to do with the dire lack of iodine in the modern diet? A survey carried out by the University of Sydney in 2006 on schoolchildren found that 59 per cent were not getting enough iodine in their diet.[139]

People with histamine headaches are advised not only to think about the histamine content of their food, but also to ensure that they have adequate iodine levels.

Serotonin

Serotonin was identified more than 50 years ago as a chemical that caused blood vessels to contract. Later, its role as a neurotransmitter was identified. One of the effects of the medications known as the triptans is to mimic serotonin and prevent nerve endings from releasing proteins associated with pain (see Chapter 9).

Fluctuating levels of serotonin have been noted in cluster, migraine, and tension headaches. In fact, the events leading up to a cluster headache have been referred to as a 'serotonin storm'.

Serotonin is a neurotransmitter that we produce in our bodies from another dietary amino acid, tryptophan, after it has gone through a reaction to produce hydroxytryptamine, or 5-HT. As the precursor to serotonin, 5-HT is often used in discussion to stand for serotonin.

Serotonin is synthesised in mast cells and nerve endings, and stored in platelets in the bloodstream. The reaction requires folic acid as a catalyst.

The neurotransmitter can be classified — along with melatonin, dopamine, adrenalin, and nor-adrenalin — as a 'phenolic amine' (see Chapter 12). Chemically speaking, this group is also 'monoamine'. Most people know about serotonin because of the popularity of the antidepressants known as selective serotonin re-uptake inhibitors (SSRIs). The best known of this family is Prozac. These medications are believed to relieve depression by blocking the body's routine breakdown of naturally produced serotonin.

Among the worst outcomes of the use of SSRIs is the serotonergic syndrome, a condition marked by agitation, hypertension, headache, raised body temperature, sweating, nausea, and diarrhoea. (This is comparable to the hypertensive crisis discussed under 'tyramine' in Chapter 12.) The serotonergic syndrome is most commonly seen when the SSRI interacts adversely with other medications or drugs (notably MAOIs), opioids, and cocaine. However, it is sometimes seen when SSRIs interact with some of nature's molecules, such as components from St John's Wort, ginseng, and nutmeg. The combination of prescription medications and street drugs causes great diagnostic difficulties, and sometimes life-threatening situations in the emergency room.

A little-known fact about serotonin is that up to 90 per cent of it is produced in the gut. Its many functions include the modulation of mood and pain, and it is also important for the regulation of appetite. There are many more serotonin receptors in the gut than there are in the brain, and this is one of the reasons that the gut is often referred to as the 'second brain'. So it should not surprise us that for migraine, cluster, and tension headaches, gut symptoms such as nausea and vomiting are known accompaniments. Some migraineurs report that the very act of vomiting (sometimes self-induced) significantly relieves a migraine attack.

We can also see why both selective and non-selective serotonin re-uptake *inhibitors* have been tried for most of these kinds of headaches. Dysfunction of the control systems for serotonin is part of the headache story generally, and does not seem to be confined to migraine. Serotonin is certainly abundant in the nerve endings around the cerebral blood vessels. It has been found repeatedly in migraine (both MA and MO) that plasma serotonin levels are elevated *during* attacks, but fall below average levels *between* attacks.[140] This makes sense in terms of the use of triptans. You have to use them early, presumably while the levels are still low. If the serotonin has started to surge, the addition of more serotonin effects is unlikely to help, and indeed, may lead to some unpleasant side effects.

There is more on 5-HT in Chapter 9 and on serotonergic effects in Chapter 10.

Serotonin and sex

Chapter 4 discussed 'sexual headaches', and showed that the relationship between sex and headache is not simple. Here is a study that looks more closely at that matter. In 2006, a research team led by Timothy Houle in Chicago looked at the relationship between self-rated sexual desire and headache. The subjects were either college students or young adults from the local community recruited on the basis of suffering at least ten headaches a year. They were divided into groups — either migraine or tension-type headache — based on the current diagnostic criteria of the International Headache Society.

The migraineurs reported higher levels of sexual desire. When the researchers considered possible mechanisms, this made sense to them. It has been shown that the serotonin precursor 5-HT has a complex relationship with migraine, including involvement in the initiation, onset, and termination of an attack. It is also known that migraine sufferers have low levels of circulating 5-HT.

The researchers commented that other research has shown that an *excess* of 5-HT in the 'mating centre' in the midbrain inhibits the effect of testosterone, and therefore reduces libido. Moreover, the side effects of SSRIs, also connected with serotonin, include loss of libido and the inhibition of orgasm. The researchers conjectured that individual differences between subjects, and a predictable difference between males and females in the scores for sexual desire, related to variations in 5-HT receptor sub-types and to other neuroendocrine differences whose role in sexual desire remains unknown.[141]

NEUROPEPTIDE NEUROTRANSMITTERS

We have just looked at some small-molecule neuro-transmitters. Here are some other types of neurotransmitters.

- angiotensin II
- beta-endorphin
- bradykinin
- corticotropin
- corticotropin-releasing hormone
- neurotensin
- somatostatin
- Substance P
- vasopressin.

Our main interest is in Substance P. It seems that the transmission of the pain message from the brainstem to higher up the chain depends on the release of the chemical known as Substance P. This neuropeptide is found throughout the brain and the spinal cord, and is accepted to be important in pain transmission. It has the effect of exciting nerve cells, and is known to increase glutamate activity in the nervous system. It is involved in the awareness of pain (nociception), inflammation, and — interestingly — mood disorders.

Substance P has specific receptors, known as NK1 receptors, and these are often found in association with the 5-HT (serotonin) receptors. Substance P antagonists have been studied for their effects in pain modulation and mood disorders. Capsaicin (an alkaloid found in capsicums) is a known antagonist to Substance P and has a proven pain-modulation effect.

Because Substance P plays a role in both hormone sensitivity and sexual function, it is one piece in the puzzle of 'hormonal headaches' and 'sexual headaches'.

Molecules with neurotransmitter and neuromodulator function

The lists above are not complete. As we have seen, other molecules, such as nitric oxide, can act as neurotransmitters. There are also neuromodulators. These are any molecule — whether produced within the body or found (for example, in food) — that might have an effect on nerve transmission.

We looked at salicylates, amines, and tyramine in Chapter 12. Some other molecules with neurotransmitter or neuro-modulator function are:

- **Homocysteine:** Recent genetic work has highlighted homocysteine for its role in the pain cascade. Chapter 2 looked at this in the discussion of the MTHFR gene. High levels of homocysteine are associated with cardiovascular disease and Alzheimer's, and are known to produce endothelial cell damage. (The endothelium is the layer of cells lining hollow organs in the body, such as the stomach or blood vessels.) When endothelial cells suffer damage, an enzyme in the endothelial cells known as nitric oxide synthase releases nitric oxide (more on that shortly).

- **Calcitonin gene-related peptide (CGRP):** This protein is found in the peripheral and central nervous systems, and, most significantly, in the trigeminal ganglion. It has been researched for its connection to pain in migraine and most other headaches (see Chapter 3). CGRP seems to 'wind up' the nerve endings, increasing their sensitivity to pain.

Both genetic factors and the triptan medications influence its action.

- **Nitric oxide:** This is a very simple molecule consisting of one atom of nitrogen and one of oxygen. It is an important signalling molecule in mammals, and plays a significant role in neuroscience and immunology. As a result, it was named the 'Molecule of the Year' in 1992. The enzyme NOS produces nitric oxide by acting on an amino acid called L-arginine. The popular drug Viagra works by releasing nitric oxide. L-arginine is nature's Viagra.

For those interested in the chemistry of all of this, Diagram 1 (page 50) and Diagram 7 (page 310) may be helpful.

If we look at Diagram 1, we see that the metabolism of arginine has a direct impact on the pathways of microglial activation and neuronal damage. We can also observe that glutamate and aspartate are part of this cycle.

The artificial sweetener aspartame releases the excitatory aspartate during digestion. Large amounts may have undesirable consequences. Diagrams 1 and 7 show where this enzyme works. Aspartame has been shown to increase glutamate toxicity and, indeed, has been described as the 'worst of the NMDA toxins in our food', with MSG (glutamate), named as a co-toxin. Through an increase in peroxynitrite, leading to glial damage, aspartame has been suggested as a possible link to an increasing number of conditions, including Parkinson's disease, multiple sclerosis, brain tumours, mental illness, learning and behavioural disorders, autism, and dementia. If this 'allowed' food additive warns us by giving us a headache, we should regard our headaches as serving a very valuable function indeed.[142]

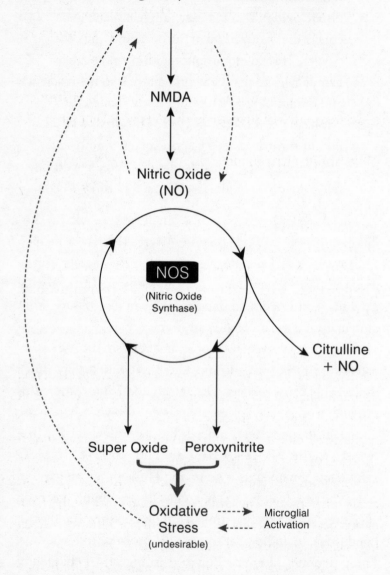

Diagram 7: Nitric oxide chemistry and NMDA sensitivity

The gene for NOS is polymorphic. If you got a double dose of a particular vulnerable polymorphism of this gene — one from each parent — then aspartame may cause you to be ill. These polymorphisms may also explain why some men get headaches when they use Viagra. Certain polymorphisms have been shown to be linked to other medical conditions. Notably, one version, known as eNOS asp298, is strongly associated with MA, hypertension, and pre-eclampsia.

More about nitric oxide

As we have just seen, nitric oxide is a signalling molecule. It supports a healthy interaction between blood vessels, platelets, and white cells known as macrophages, which operate at sites of damage, such as epithelial cells (blood-vessel linings). The release of nitric oxide increases blood flow to a site of injury. The downside of this for the headache sufferer is the throbbing headache and pain during a headache event.

The effects of nitric oxide are complicated and confusing. It has often been implicated in the migraine cascade. It is also closely linked to cluster headaches, tension headaches, and 'histamine headaches'. Histamine, too, can cause a release of nitric oxide from the endothelium.

Another clue is glyceryl tri-nitrate (GTN), a mainstay in the treatment of angina. We know that GTN works by releasing nitric oxide to relax blood vessels. But GTN can cause migraine-type headaches, and people who suffer from cluster headaches usually avoid it for this reason. Furthermore, GTN can trigger paroxysmal hemicrania.[143]

So it is reasonable to conclude that nitric oxide plays a role in various 'unrelated' headaches.

But just when we think that we are getting a handle on all this, a new suggestion comes up. The homocysteine research mentioned above suggests that blood-vessel linings damaged by high levels of homocysteine may in fact have *reduced* capacity to produce nitric oxide. The authors of one study hypothesise that some of the symptoms of the migraine attack, not to mention the increased risk of stroke in migraineurs, may stem from *low levels* of nitric oxide.[144]

It is best simply to conclude that research on nitric oxide will contribute to our understanding of what goes on in our brains during a headache. No further research is needed for us to conclude that too much is as problematic as too little.

Summary

We can say that molecules such as homocysteine and nitric oxide have a role in various headache types. Appropriate levels of these at the right times and in the right places are part of a healthy physiological response. It is instructive to refer to the migraine cascade, and to bear in mind its potential relevance to other kinds of headache. No doubt new research will unravel the minutiae of headache sequences. My experience is that the solutions can be a whole lot simpler than trying to manipulate this complex chemistry.

THE RECEPTORS

On the whole, the molecules we have just been discussing exert their effects by docking on a matching receptor site.

In doing so, they may act as an inhibitor or an excitor, either reducing or encouraging a reaction. Any one transmitter may have more than one compatible receptor site. The same molecule, therefore, may have a different effect, depending on the receptor site to which it has attached.

For instance, acetylcholine is a neurotransmitter that we met in Chapter 11, which acts in both the sympathetic and the parasympathetic nervous systems. As a generalisation, it activates nicotinic receptors in the sympathetic nervous system or muscarinic receptors in the parasympathetic. Depending on which of the two types it activates, the effects are quite different.

But it is not only the messenger molecules that vary in their effects. Some receptor sites act 'promiscuously' and accept a range of messenger molecules. The behaviour of the receptor differs according to which molecule is activating it. This phenomenon, confusing to lay people (and often to the medically trained, too), is another example of the efficiencies built into nature's biological systems.

Receptor sites tend to fall into one of two classifications, either fast or slow. The technical names are 'ligand-gated receptors' and 'G-protein receptors'. When a fast receptor is activated, it opens an ion channel and allows the influx of potassium ions (positively charged) and chloride ions (negatively charged). The net effect of these electrical charges may either excite or inhibit the nerve cell in question.

Glutamate and aspartate have a stimulatory effect on the slow receptors. Slow receptors are indirectly linked to ion channels via a second messenger system. They cannot be characterised as either 'inhibitory' or 'excitatory'. The influence of the receptor accords with the particular neurotransmitter activating it.

Receptors can be classified in groups according to which neurotransmitters they respond to: serotonin responsive (serotinergic), nor-adrenalin responsive, dopamine responsive (dopaminergic), and acetylcholine responsive (cholinergic). The location of these receptors varies according to which part of the body we are discussing. The effects may be vascular or behavioural, or may relate to something like 'nausea' or 'perception'.

There are further complexities within each group of receptors. For instance, the serotonergic receptors are subdivided according to their precursor as 5-HT 1, 5-HT 2, 5-HT 3, and so on. These can be classed into sub-subgroups signified by capital letters. Thus the 5-HT 1 receptors are named from 'A' to 'F'. The drug Sumatriptan acts as an agonist at the 5-HT 1B and 5-HT 1D receptors, while ergotamine acts as a partial agonist at these sites. At same time, ergotamine acts as an antagonist at 1D receptors. The new triptan, Zolmitriptan, acts as an agonist at 1D, but does not act at 1B. By contrast, methysergide acts as an antagonist at 5-HT 2 receptors, or at least at those classified as 2A, C, and D.

You can see that it is all very complicated — and that is still only a small part of the story.

Adenosine receptors

We met these receptors in Chapter 10, when discussing migraine-prone rats. The rats turned out to be extremely sensitive to alcohol, and were relieved by taking caffeine or aspirin. Humans have four types of adenosine receptor, and each is regulated by a separate gene.

Two of the adenosine receptors have important roles in the brain, regulating the release of neurotransmitters such as dopamine and glutamate. In the case of one of the receptors, a particular polymorphism (of the A2A gene) has been associated with migraine with aura.[145] We might guess that the migrainous rats have inherited a similar set of receptors.

It is the job of adenosine receptors to block the release of acetylcholine. Caffeine stops them from doing this, and thus allows acetylcholine production to go ahead. Acetate, from alcohol breakdown, does the opposite. In this scenario, acetylcholine relieves the headache. So caffeine is beneficial, especially after an alcohol-induced headache, because it counteracts the blocking action of the adenosine receptors.

It is possible that headaches associated with glutamate in the diet could be similarly helped by caffeine. As we saw in Chapter 3, glutamate release is a key player in the headache event. It is caffeine's interaction with adenosine receptors that results in your headache being relieved by a cup of coffee, or a pill with caffeine in it. However, as with any chemical that affects brain chemistry, the reaction may be different for different people, and the question of dependence must always be considered.

Finally, the A2A receptor is under investigation for its possible role in insomnia, pain, depression, drug addiction, and Parkinson's disease. Both caffeine craving and caffeine sensitivity have been noted in connection with these various conditions.

NMDA receptors

Current research indicates that the receptors for N-methyl-D-aspartic acid (NMDA) play an important role in the mechanisms of migraine. We met them in Chapter 11 in the context of multiple chemical sensitivity and complex regional pain syndrome.

The NMDA receptor is described as a 'glutamate-regulated ion channel that regulates excitatory synaptic transmission'. That is quite a mouthful, but it just means that glutamate sensitivity is played out through this receptor. As there are various polymorphisms for the NMDA receptor, the genes that you inherit for this receptor play a role in your sensitivity to environmental chemicals.[146]

Nociceptive receptors

'Nociceptive' means 'causing or relating to pain', so this term refers to pain receptors. Any noxious stimulus, such as excessive heat or pressure, activates these receptors.

The message of pain is carried from the receptor, into the spinal cord, and up to the brain. There are both fast and slow nerve fibres. They ascend the spinal column in different tracts, after interacting with intermediate neurons. The fast fibres relay the message, which is 'perceived' by the cortex within a fraction of a second. Thus, the pain is quickly and accurately located. The slow fibres terminate in different places throughout the brainstem. The pain is poorly located, and can be described as 'aching', 'throbbing', or 'burning'.

All nociceptive experience is subject to the body's inbuilt analgesic systems. These include nociceptive inhibitory neurons in the spinal cord, and the loop though the PAG matter that we discussed in Chapter 12.

GATE CONTROL

Gate control is a term that describes the provision of an independent stimulus at the same time as pain, so that the painful experience is modified by the other, less noxious stimulus. Doctors often rub the arm of a child both before and after an injection, as if to distract the brain from the painful experience. We all tend to rub the affected part when we have hurt ourselves. Therapy for complex regional pain syndrome involves tapping or rubbing the painful spot. Headache sufferers often rub their temples or forehead. Tiger Balm ointment (discussed in Chapter 9) also uses the principles of gate control.

Opioid receptors

These receptors, which occur throughout the body, are activated by the body's production of endorphins. They are part of the pain-control system, and people have varying capacity to invoke such control. The 'runner's high' is an extreme example of exercise as a means of inducing endorphin production. Other examples are meditation and other mind–body control exercises.

Toll-like receptors

Toll-like receptors are relative newcomers to discussions of everyday medical issues.[147] Named for the 'toll' gene, which was first identified in the late 1980s in fruit flies, toll-like receptors were recognised in the late 1990s. They are found on the surface of a cell in everything from bacteria and plants through to complex beings such as humans. They are key regulators of both adaptive and innate immune responses.

As part of humans' immune defence, we have receptors designed to recognise foreign molecules, such as those on the surface of microbes, and parasites like worms. This is part of the conversation between certain key immune cells (called dendritic cells) and the outside world. Toll-like receptors are able to recognise a molecule as foreign, and their job is to help decide whether it poses a threat to the organism. These toll-like receptors can be fast (ligand-gated), but they may also communicate by altering the signalling in slow (G-protein) receptors in dendritic cells.[148]

In regard to headache, the importance of these toll-like receptors is their presence on glial cells (discussed in Chapter 11) and their ability to recognise a range of molecules — from heat-shock proteins (such as gluten) to opioids. Opiates and opioid substances, you will remember, are alkaloids. Gluten (as gluteomorphin), casein from milk (caseomorphin), and eggs all have some opiate activity. Specifically, many of the foods that are implicated in migraine have alkaloid or opiate activity, including citrus and tomatoes. A colleague of mine has tried the opiate blocker Naltrexone in a couple of resistant migraineurs with considerable success. Along with the drug, he also restricts and rotates the intakes of these foods.[149]

How does this relate to me?

I have told you about molecules and their receptors not to confuse you but to make some important points. Although the complexity of the receptors really belongs to neurologists and drug researchers, G-protein receptors are involved in many illnesses, and are the target of approximately one-third of all modern drugs. The types of G-protein receptors you possess may help to explain why you get the headaches you do.

The genetic variations in receptor types create another way by which you might react badly to different medications or environmental toxins (such as perfumes, paints, and additives) generally regarded as 'safe'. If you are one of the people who react badly to many medications, then, as was the case with the varying CYP polymorphisms that control phase-1 enzymes (see Chapter 11), your G-protein genetics may possibly explain why. You are not just being contrary. We might reasonably regard you as having multiple chemical sensitivity. It is a bitter irony that the people most in need of medicines may be the very ones who benefit least, or get the most side effects.[150]

CHEMISTRY: SOME LOOSE ENDS

As we draw to a close the story of chemistry in headache, here are some other chemical facts. Some of them I find fascinating, and all of them tell us something about the causes of headaches and point to possible solutions. Let us start with Lydia.

Lydia's story

Lydia's mother accompanied her to her consultation with me. In her late twenties, Lydia was painfully thin, and my first reaction was to think that she must be suffering from cancer or an eating disorder. Her symptoms included muscle wasting, weakness, spasms in the limbs, and headache. She also had poor circulation: she was wearing a heavy coat in temperate weather. A specialist had ordered blood tests, but the results showed no evidence of obvious pathology. She had been diagnosed with polymyalgia rheumatica and given steroids. An alternative diagnosis of possible early multiple sclerosis was also under consideration. The specialist had ordered an MRI, but had found no evidence of typical MS lesions.

Lydia was a bright university graduate, and her research on the internet had left her dissatisfied with her diagnosis. I took an extensive dietary history and was stunned to find that she was drinking about three litres of diet cola, which is sweetened with aspartame, a day. For any such patient, I would run some tests. One of them is a special test for vitamin B12 — in the form of 'active B12', or holotranscobalamin. Her regular vitamin B12 level was well within the normal range. Her *active* B12, however, was the lowest I had ever seen — about one-quarter of the minimal effective level.

I gave her two shots of vitamin B12: regular B12 in one arm, and methyl B12 in the other. I used the methylated form of B12 because I know that this is the form required by the central nervous system. The methylated forms gets across the blood–brain barrier. It is a key nutrient in the maintenance of the myelin sheaths, and I have given it to MS patients many times. Even though the MRI showed no de-myelination in Lydia's brain or nervous system, her body was behaving as if it were happening. Only later did I piece it together and appreciate the role that methyl B12 plays in protecting the nervous system from aspartame, glutamate, and nitric oxide. All of these excitatory molecules are implicated in the pathology of degenerative brain disorders such as Parkinson's, Alzheimer's, and circulation disorders.

Among the other tests I ordered for Lydia was MTHFR genotyping (explained in Chapter 2). Like me, she had a double dose of the polymorphism that is least desirable when it comes to circulation and headache. My guess is that she not only had the methylation defect that goes with this genotype, but also NOS or MTR/R polymorphisms, which require more than average support from folate and vitamins B6 and B12. She certainly was not getting enough to meet the demands placed on her biochemistry by the massive consumption of aspartame in the diet cola.

By giving up this drink (which was not easy at first), and taking supplementary B vitamins (including a few more injections), she brought about a complete resolution of all of her symptoms, including her headaches.

A few months later, I was discussing Lydia's story with a colleague. She told me of an almost identical case of a patient diagnosed with 'atypical multiple sclerosis'. This patient also recovered when she was persuaded to cease her daily intake of two to three litres of diet cola.

Both of us wondered why *anyone* would want to drink that much. But when you consider that aspartame is an excitatory molecule in the central nervous system, the word 'addictive' seems to apply.

Methylation

Lydia's story is a simple clinical example of addiction, but it also shows us something about methylation. Chapter 2 described the effects of folic acid and other B-group vitamins in headaches (and other conditions), as a result of interaction with genes such as the MTHFR variants.

Less commonly known is another role that folic acid has in *most* of our genes. It seems to have an epigenetic effect, modifying genetic information through environmental influences. The DNA does not change, but the expression of the genes does. An epigenetic effect resembles a dimmer control on a light switch; it may turn the gene down, or even turn it off. If this dimmer switch is acting on genes for inflammation or cancer, it will be useful. But if we lack folic acid in our diet, or have a variant of the MTHFR gene that reduces our ability to handle dietary folic acid, we are at a disadvantage. Perhaps we need more folic acid than other people. We certainly need more than a diet high in heavily processed foods will give us. Poor diets have led authorities in some nations to fortify bread with folic acid. This move has been controversial, for reasons that we will look at in a minute.

The biochemical function of folic acid is to act as a 'methyl donor'. This means that it donates a methyl group to certain chemical substrates so that they become something else. The action is known as methylation. We have just seen the benefit of giving vitamin B12, itself a methyl donor, in a methylated form. Other methyl donors include vitamin B6 and s-adenosyl methionine (SAMe). SAMe is often referred to as the body's 'universal methyl donor'.

You will be wondering what a methyl group is, and the

answer is deceptively simple: it is a carbon atom with three hydrogen atoms stuck on it. But although the methyl group that is passed around is simple, the role of methylation in biology cannot be overstated. Methylation plays a critical role in many important reactions — for example, the conversion of dietary tryptophan to serotonin, and the conversion of dietary tyrosine to dopamine. But it does not stop there. Look back at Diagram 1, on page 50. When a methyl group from the folic acid cycle is transferred into the SAMe cycle, it rescues homocysteine from accumulating and converts it back to methionine. The methyl group on methionine now gets sent out for the repair and synthesis of RNA and DNA, among other things, and the whole cycle starts again.

So methyl groups have many important functions, and the epigenetic effect is one of the most significant of these. Methylation of a gene tends to turn the gene down — it reduces its effect. Recent research suggests that men who take folic acid supplements may be more at risk from prostate cancer.[151] This research is not well supported, and it seems to defy previous research about folic acid in cancer, but in theory prostate cancer could be *more* likely to develop if the folic acid turns down a tumour-suppressing gene. Hence the controversy over adding folic acid to commonly eaten foods such as bread.

Headaches as 'ion channelopathies'

Chapter 2, looking at the various genes associated with migraine, showed that many of these genes manifest themselves in the balancing act between nutrients such as calcium and magnesium or sodium and potassium. You may have a genetic inheritance that finds it difficult to achieve this balancing act. Mild gene 'defects' may not be able to handle dietary imbalances, and thus we get sick. This is what we mean by an 'ion channelopathy'. Many headache variants are now regarded as a problem in the ion channels, and are known as inherited ion channelopathies. We have just discussed the role of NMDA receptors in migraine and chemical sensitivity, and we saw that they are 'glutamate-regulated ion channels'.

Ion channels

Every cell in the body — indeed, every organelle within each cell — is wrapped in a membrane. Built into the structure of the membrane are pores, made up of special proteins. These pores are there to let small particles known as ions through the membrane. The pores are called channels.

It is via these channels in the cell membranes that nerve and muscle cells send and receive their messages. The channels are activated either by a small electrical current or by a transmitter molecule. When an atom carrying an electrical charge goes through a channel, it activates it, and is said to be 'voltage-activated'. Examples of these charged atoms include calcium ions and sodium ions. They are represented as Ca^{++} and Na^{+}, with the plus sign indicating a positive charge.

The shape of the pore or channel is an inherited characteristic. We all inherit channels of greater or less efficiency for each channel type. Other examples of channels include the potassium channel and the chloride channel. Elements that look like the ones for which the channel was 'designed' often function as the counterbalancing force; thus, magnesium can moderate calcium, and potassium can moderate sodium. A new science of channelopathies is emerging, whereby certain illnesses can be attributed to the inheritance of a particular channel. Familial hemiplegic migraine can be regarded as a channelopathy (calcium channel), as can cystic fibrosis (chloride channel), and also the cardiac problem of Long QT syndrome (various channels, including potassium and sodium).

As our understanding of these channelopathies increases, future genetic testing will help us to design diet and nutrient programs to help manage headaches and many other hereditary tendencies to illness. For the moment, it seems safest to stick to a primitive diet that preserves nature's appropriate nutrient balance.

Vomiting

Vomiting is a complex business, with many pathways and receptors involved. The purpose, we can assume, is to eject poisonous substances from the stomach before they can do us serious harm. Vomiting is a significant part of many headaches, and, as we have already discussed, vomiting (like sex) can sometimes relieve a headache.

We saw in Chapter 7 that migraine is recognised as one of the risk factors for severe vomiting in pregnancy. For a pregnant woman, there is clear value in becoming sensitive to poisonous food (or noxious gases). Similarly, vomiting after a head injury warns that dangerous pressure may be building up in the brain. But when vomiting becomes a common part of headaches, what is nature trying to tell us?

Are we being warned that we have eaten or inhaled something that is bad for us, or have the wires in our brain become crossed? I think that various factors are at work, sensitising our nerve endings to all sort of things; so stress, motion sickness, rapid eye movements, and even electromagnetic fields (Chapter 4) can trigger nausea, vomiting, or a headache itself.

Let us look at what goes on in the brain when a person vomits. The vomiting centre is in the brainstem, where we find neurotransmitters such as choline, histamine, dopamine, serotonin, and opioids, along with their various receptors. Activation of these neurotransmitters stimulates the vomiting reflex. (Indeed, one of the undesirable effects of the opioid morphine is nausea and vomiting.) So a lot can be going on, with the interaction of neurochemistry, especially serotonin receptors, the vagus nerve, and the effects of meditation and drugs such as the very effective ondansetron.[152]

Before we move on, let's mention another neurotransmitter. Our old friend Substance P and its receptors are in high concentrations in the vomiting centre. Considering the roles that Substance P plays in pain and mood, a link between pain, mood, and vomiting is not improbable. It looks as if, whatever the original stimulus that caused the vomiting, Substance P may be the main regulatory factor. Little wonder that pharmacologists are researching drugs that can block Substance P.

I wrote this chapter to look at the chemistry of headache in more detail — in particular, the chemistry of the neurotransmitters and the receptors that they act upon. Once, words such as 'neurotransmitter' or 'methylator' were the domain of the biochemist or the neurologist. That has changed. They have entered the everyday language of many, and are commonly used by the patients I see. I think that this is a good thing, and I have tried to contribute to this understanding.

Conclusion

'Listen to the patient; he is telling you the diagnosis.'
Sir William Osler

Throughout this book, I have tried to outline the science behind headaches, and by that means to suggest simple strategies for dealing with them. We know the enormous burden that headache places on Western society. Although I have no hard evidence, I'm certain that headache was much less troublesome in earlier societies, and that 'primitive' societies had little in the way of primary headache at all.

Mother Nature did not intend for one in six of us to need regular medication just to function. Headache sufferers should see themselves as canaries in the mine in an increasingly toxic world. We have a choice: we can lament our genetic susceptibility and spend a good part of our income propping up the pharmaceutical industry; or we can modify our diet, environment, and lifestyle. We are so busily rushing through our modern world that we have lost the capacity to look, observe, and think about what is happening around us.

I apply that to my own profession as much as to any of us as individuals. For years, patients have been telling us about their headaches. As doctors, we need to listen to them, and not just to help them choose the best drug for the problem. As a society, we need to encourage doctors to spend more time with patients, not penalise them for doing so. The current healthcare system often falls short in this regard.

Sir William Osler, sometimes called the father of modern medicine, is known for his many wise sayings. I began this book with a quote from him, and so it seems fitting to end with one, perhaps the wisest of all his sayings. I remember learning this from my teachers in my early days of medical school. I wonder how many medical students today, their heads mired in technology and their eyes glued to the computer screen, are taught this?

Now, let's conclude with an excerpt from this particularly apt poem by the Australian poet John Shaw Neilson.

The Orange Tree

The young girl stood beside me. I
Saw not what her young eyes could see:
— A light, she said, not of the sky
Lives somewhere in the Orange Tree.

— Is it , I said, of east or west?
The heartbeat of a luminous boy
Who with his faltering flute confessed
Only the edges of his joy?

Was he, I said, borne to the blue
In a mad escapade of Spring
Ere he could make a fond adieu
To his love in the blossoming?

— Listen! the young girl said. There calls
No voice, no music beats on me;
But it is almost sound: It falls
This evening on the Orange Tree.

Does he, I said, so fear the Spring
Ere the white sap too far can climb?
See in the full gold evening
All happenings of the olden time?

Is he so goaded by the green?
Does the compulsion of the dew
Make him unknowable but keen
Asking with beauty of the blue?

— Listen! The young girl said. For all
Your hapless talk you fail to see
There is a light, a step, a call,
This evening on the Orange Tree.

Appendix 1: Food Groups

This list is confined to plant foods. Every living creature that has ever has walked, crawled, flown, hopped, or swum has at some stage been eaten by some other creature, and so a complete taxonomy of the animal world is not necessary here. It might be useful to consider, however, that many creatures that we consider as pests are consumed rather than poisoned in other cultures. These include grubs, larvae, locusts, and other insects, and even deep-fried tarantulas.

Actinidiaceae: Chinese gooseberry or kiwifruit (*Actinidia chinensis*)

Algae: agar-agar, carrageen, dulse, kelp, or seaweed

Alliaceae: chives, garlic, leek, onion, shallot (all *Allium* species)

Amaranthaceae: Chinese spinach or hinn choi (*Amaranthus tricolor*), grain amaranth (A. *hypochondriacus*), green amaranth (A. *viridis*)

Araucariaceae: bunya nuts (*Araucaria bidwilli*)

Arrowroot family, *Marantaceae*: arrowroot (*Maranta arundinacea*)

Arum family, *Araceae*: ceriman (*Monstera*), dasheen (*Colocasia*), taro, malanga, yautia

Asclepiadaceae: bush banana (*Leichhardtia australis, Marsdenia vividiflora*) — leaves, flowers, tubers

Banana family, *Musaceae*: arrowroot (*Musa*), banana, plantain

Basellaceae: creeping spinach or basella (*Basella alba*), ulluco (*Ullucus tuberosa*)

Beech family, *Fagaceae*: chestnut (*Castanea sativa*), dwarf chestnut or chinquapin

Birch family, *Betulaceae*: hazelnut or filbert (*Corylus avellana*), oil of birch (wintergreen)

Bombacaceae: durian fruit (*Durio zibethinus*)

Borage family, *Boraginaceae* (herbs): borage, comfrey (leaf and root)

Buckwheat family, *Polygonaceae*: buckwheat (*Fagopyrum esculentum*), garden sorrel, rhubarb (stems only), sea grape

Buttercup family, *Ranunculaceae*: golden seal

Cactus family, *Cactaceae*: prickly pear

Canna family, *Cannaceae*: Queensland arrowroot

Caper family, *Capparidaceae*: caper

Carpetweed family, *Aizoaceae*: Warragul greens (*Tetragonia tetragniodes*), various pigface (*Carpobrutus* species)

Carrot family, *Umbelliferae* a.k.a. *Apiaceae*: angelica, anise, carraway, carrot, celeriac, celery, chervil, coriander, cumin, dill, fennel, gotu kola, lovage, parsley, parsnip, sweet cicely, skirret

Cashew family, *Anacardiaceae*: burdekin plum (*Pleiogynium timorense*), cashew, mango, pistachio

Citrus family, *Rutaceae*: lime, lemon, orange, grapefruit, citron (*Citrus* and *Microcitrus* species); cumquat (*Fortunella* species)

Combretaceae: kakadu plum (*Terminalia ferdinandiana*), native almond (*T. grandiflora*), nut tree (*T. arostrata*), sea almond (*T. catappa*)

Composite family, *Compositae* a.k.a. *Asteraceae*: alpine yam daisy, boneset, burdock root, cardoon, chamomile, chicory or endive, coltsfoot, costmary, dandelion, escarole, globe artichoke, goldenrod, Jerusalem artichoke, lettuce, pyrethrum, romaine, safflower, salsify, santolina, scolymus (Spanish oyster plant), scorzonera, shungiku (*Chrysanthemum coronarium*), southernwood, sunflower (*Helianthus annus*), tansy, tarragon, witloof chicory or French endive, wormwood (absinthe), yam daisy, yarrow

Conifer family, *Gramineae*: juniper (gin), pine nut (pi-on)

Custard-apple family, *Annona* species: custard-apple, papaw or pawpaw

Cyatheaceae: soft tree fern (*Dicksonia antarctica*)

Cycad family, *Coniferae*: cycad seed (*Cycas media*), Florida arrowroot (*Zamia*)

Davidsoniaceae: Davidson's plum (*Davidsonia pruriens*)

Ebony family, *Ebonaceae*: persimmons (Japanese and American), black plum, date plum (all *Diospyros* species)

Flax family, *Linaceae*: flaxseed

Fungi, *Agaricaceae*: yeasts, moulds, mushrooms, truffles

Ginger family, *Zingiberaceae*: cardamon, East Indian arrowroot (*Curcuma*), ginger, turmeric

Ginseng family, *Araliaceae*: American ginseng, Chinese ginseng

Goosefoot family, *Chenopodiaceae*: beetroot, chard, quinoa, silverbeet, spinach, sugar beet, tampala

Gourd family, *Cucurbitaceae*: bitter melon, choko, cucumber, gherkin, squashes (butternut etc.), pumpkins, sweet melons (cantaloupe etc.), watermelons, zucchini

Grape family, *Vitaceae*: grapes, raisins, wine, wine vinegar, brandy

Grass family, *Gramineae* a.k.a. *Poaceae*: barley (*Hordenum vulgare*), corn (*Zea mays*), millet, oats, rice, sorghum, triticale, wheat, bamboo shoots, sugarcane, lemongrass, wild rice, woollybutt grass (*Eragrostis eriopoda*)

Heath family, *Ericaceae*: bearberry, blueberry, cranberry, huckleberry, tree strawberry (*Arbutus unedo*)

Honeysuckle family, *Caprifoliaceae*: elderberry

Horsetail family, *Equisetaceae*: shavegrass (horsetail)

Iris family, *Iridaceae*: orris root, saffron (*Crocus*)

Lamiaceae: bush tea leaf (*Ocimum tenuiflorum*), hairy basil (*O. americanum*)

Laurel family, *Lauraceae*: avocado, bay leaf, cassia bark, cinnamon

Legume family, *Leguminoseae*, a.k.a. *Fabaceae*: alfalfa (sprouts), beans (numerous varieties), soybeans, peas (numerous varieties), peanuts, lentils, carob, fenugreek, jicama tubers, tamarind

Lily family, *Liliaceae*: Aloe vera, asparagus, bulbine lily or wild onion (*Bulbine bulbosa*), chocolate lily or grass lily (*Dichopogon strictus*)

Linden family, *Tiliaceae*: basswood or linden, melokhia (*Corchorus olitorius*)

Madder family, *Rubiaceae*: coffee (*Coffea arabica*, *C. canephora*), woodruff

Mallow family, *Malvaceae*: althea root, cottonseed oil, roselle or rosella (*Hibiscus sabdariffa*), okra (*H. esculentus*)

Malpighia family, *Malpighiaceae*: acerola (Barbados cherry)

Maple family: sap of sugar maple (*Acer saccharum*)

Mint family, *Labiatae* (herbs): various mints, basil, bergamot, catnip, chinese artichoke, clary, dittany, horehound, hyssop, lavender, lemon balm, marjoram, oregano, pennyroyal, perilla, rosemary, sage, summer savory, thyme, winter savory

Morning-glory family, *Convolvulaceae*: bush potato (*Ipomoea costata*), sweet potato (*I. batatas*), kangkong (*I. aquatica*)

Mulberry family, *Moraceae*: breadfruit (*Artocarpus incisa*), various figs (*Ficus* species), jackfruit, mulberry

Mustard family, a.k.a. Cabbage family, *Cruciferae* a.k.a. *Brassicaceae*: various rockets (*Cakile* species, *Heperis* species, *Eruca* species), broccoli, brussels sprouts, cabbage, watercress, canola, cauliflower, cress, horseradish, kale, kohlrabi, mizuna, komatsuna, radish, rutabaga, turnip

Myrtle family, *Myrtaceae*:
- nectar: various bottlebrush (*Callistemon* species)
- fruit: lilly pilly, brush cherry, durobby (*Szygium* species), myrtles (*Austromyrtus* species)
- edible sap: cider gum (*Eucalyptus gunnii*)

Nasturtium family, *Tropaeolaceae*: nasturtium

Nutmeg family, *Myristicaceae*: nutmeg

Olive family, *Oleaceae*: olive (green or ripe)

Orchid family, *Orchidaceae*: vanilla

Oxalis family, *Oxalidaceae*: carambola or star fruit (*Averrhoa carambola*), oxalis or oca (*Oxalis tuberosa*)

Palm family, *Palmaceae*: coconut (*Cocos nucifera*), date, palm cabbage, sago palm

Papaya family, *Caricaceae*: papaya

Passion Flower family, *Passifloraceae*: granadilla or passion fruit

Pedalium family, *Pedaliaceae*: sesame (*Sesamum indicum*)

Pepper family, *Piperaceae*: peppercorn (*Piper* species)

Pineapple family, *Bromeliaceae*: pineapple

Pittosporaceae: appleberry (*Billardiera scandens*), purple appleberry (*B. longiflora*), sweet appleberry (*B. cymosa*)

Podocarpaceae: brown pine (*Podocarpus dispersus*), illawarra plum

(*P. elatus*), mountain plum pine (*P. lawrencei*)

Pomegranate family, *Punicaceae*: pomegranate (*Punica granatum*)

Poppy family, *Papaveraceae*: poppyseed

Potato family, a.k.a. Nightshade family, *Solanaceae*: tomato, bush tomato, tree tomato, eggplant, capsicum, chilli, potato, tobacco

Protea family, *Proteaceae*: geebungs (*Persoonia* species), bush nut (*Macadamia tetraphylla*), nectar from various banksias, grevilleas, and hakeas

Purslane family, *Portulaceae*: pigweed or purslane (*Portulaca oleracea*)

Rhamnaceae: Chinese jujube (*Zizyphus jujuba*), Indian jujube (*Z. mauritania*)

Rose family, *Rosaceae*:

- pomes: apple, azarole, crabapple, loquat, medlar, pear, quince, rosehips
- stone fruits: almond, apricot, cherry, peach (nectarine), plum (prune), sloe
- berries: blackberry, boysenberry, dewberry, loganberry, longberry, youngberry, raspberry, strawberry

Santalaceae: various ballart (*Exocarpus* species), broad-leaved native cherry (*E. latifolius*), quandong (*Santalum acuminatum*)

Sapodilla family, *Sapotaceae*: chicle (chewing gum)

Sapucaya family, *Lecythidaceae*: Brazil nut (*Bertholletia excelsa*), sapucaya nut (paradise nut)

Saxifrage family, *Saxifragaceae*: currant, gooseberry

Sedge family, *Cyperaceae*: Chinese water chestnut (*Eleocharis dulcis*), chufa (groundnut), nalgoo tuber (*Cyperus bulbosus*)

Smilacaceae: sweet tea (*Smilax glyciphylla*)

Soapberry family, *Sapindaceae*: akee apple (*Blighia sapida*), litchi or lychee, longan (*Dimocarpus longan*), rambutan (*Nephelium lappaceum*)

Spurge family, *Euphorbiaceae*: candlenut (*Aleurites moluccana*), cassava or yuca (*Manihot dulcis, M. esculenta*), castor bean

Sterculia family, *Sterculiaceae*: chocolate (cacao), cocoa, cola nut, kurrajong tree seeds

Tacca family, *Taccaceae*: Fiji arrowroot (*Tacca* species)

Tea family, *Theaceae*: tea (*Camellia sinensis*)

Valerian family, *Valerianaceae*: corn salad (*Valerianella locusta*)

Verbena family, *Verbenaceae*: lemon verbena

Walnut family, *Juglandaceae*: various walnuts (*Jugland* species), hickory nuts and pecan (*Carya* species)

Waterlily family, *Nymphaeaceae*: lotus (*Nelumbo nucifera*)

Wattle family, *Mimosaceae*: seed and edible gum or sap from various wattles (*Acacia* species), mulga (*A. aneura*)

Winteraceae: dorrigo pepper (*Tasmannia stipitata*), mountain pepper (*T. lanceolata*)

Xanthorrhoeaceae: grass tree (*Xanthorrhoea australis*)

Yam family, *Dioscoreaceae*: various types of yam (*Dioscorea* species)

Appendix 2:
Service Providers

The author cannot guarantee the accuracy of any of these laboratory tests or reliability of information they supply. The reader must take responsibility for cost, misinterpretation of results, or any other negative outcomes of any tests they undertake. Tests should always be done in conjunction with your qualified medical practitioner.

Your local pathology laboratory can provide many of the tests mentioned in this book, including some genetic tests.

GENETIC TESTING SERVICES

Some of these laboratories test internationally. Some will only release data to one of their registered practitioners. The below companies are based in the United States, the United Kingdom, or Australia, but offer their services internationally.

- Holistic Health International, www.holistichealth.com
- Metametrix, www.metametrix.com
- Fitgenes, www.fitgenes.com/77/who-is-fitgenes.aspx
- 23andMe, www.23andme.com

OTHER LABORATORIES

- Bioscreen Medical, www.bioscreenmedical.com
- Diagnostic Insight (Australia; also the Australian distributor for Metametrix), www.diagnosticinsight.com.au
- Healthscope Pathology (Australia), www.healthscopepathology.com.au
- SAFE Laboratories (Australia), www.safelabs.com.au
- Spire Healthcare (United Kingdom), www.spirehealthcare.com/spire-pathology-services

DOCTORS AND OTHER PRACTITIONERS

- Australasian College of Nutritional and Environmental Medicine, www.acnem.org (go to 'find a practitioner' for Australian and overseas practitioners)
- Australasian Integrative Medical Association, www.aima.net.au
- National Health Service Choices (United Kingdom), www.nhs.uk/Service-Search
- National Institute of Integrative Medicine (Australia), www.niim.com.au
- Health Engine (Australia), www.healthengine.com.au/find/Integrative_Medicine_Practitioner/Australia
- UK Health Care, www.ukhealthcare.uky.edu/doctors/

Further Reading

Bartley, Jim, *Healing Headaches: a New Zealand guide*, Random House, Auckland, 2007.

Bijlsma, Nicole, *Healthy Home, Healthy Family: is where you live affecting your health?*, Joshua Books, Buddina, 2012.

Buist, Robert, *Food Chemical Sensitivity: what it is and how to cope with it*, Harper & Row, Sydney, 1986.

Buist, Robert, *Food Intolerance: what it is and how to cope with it*, Collins Australia, Sydney, 1987.

D'Adamo, Peter J., *Eat Right for Your Type*, Century, New York, 2001.

Dengate, Sue, *The Failsafe Cookbook: Reducing food chemicals for calm, happy families*, Random House, Sydney, 2007.

Doidge, Norman, *The Brain that Changes Itself*, Scribe Publications, Melbourne, 2008.

Eaton, S. Boyd; Shostak, Marjorie; and Konner, Melvin, *The Stone-Age Health Programme: Diet and exercise as nature intended*, Angus & Robertson, Sydney, 1989.

Gedgadus, Nora, *Primal Body, Primal Mind: beyond the paleo diet for total health and a longer life*, www.primalbody-primalmind.com

Mellowship, Dawn, *Toxic Beauty*, Octopus Publishing Group, London, 2009.

Pall, Martin J., *Explaining Unexplained Illnesses*, Haworth Press, New York, 2007.

Royal Prince Alfred Hospital Allergy Unit, *Friendly Food: recipes for life, the essential guide to avoiding allergies, additives, and problem chemicals*, Murdoch Books, Sydney, 2002.

Smith, Rick, and Lourie, Bruce, *Slow Death by Rubber Duck: how the toxic chemistry of everyday life affects our health*, University of Queensland Press, Brisbane, 2009.

Stipanuk, Martha H., *Biochemical and Physiological Aspects of Human Nutrition*, W.B. Saunders Company, Philadelphia, 2000.

Walsh, William J., *Nutrient Power: heal your biochemistry and heal your brain*, Skyhorse Publishing, New York, 2012.

Yasko, Amy, *Genetic Bypass: using nutrition to bypass genetic mutations*, Matrix Press, 2005.

Acknowledgements

With thanks to Dr Robert Buist, who taught me how patients might manage their own headaches, and to Dr Ross Wilson, a doctor's doctor.

To the following doctors, who have helped by reading the manuscript, making comments, or who have helped me with my own health struggles: Trish and David Allen, Paul Beaumont, Ron Brookes, John Cummins, Ron Field, Simon Hammond, Annemarie Hennessy, Ross Walker, and Eric Wegman.

And inestimable thanks go to my husband, Keith; daughters, Zoe and Jocelyn; and sons, Guy and Jude, without whose input this book would never have happened.

Thanks also to all at Scribe, and to Janet Mackenzie, whose last-minute efforts again demonstrated the value of an editor in the production of a book.

Notes

1   Senior, Kathryn, 'Facts and Figures about Headache', *Headache Expert*, 19 June 2012, www.headacheexpert.co.uk/facts-figures-about-headaches.html

2   'National Headache Foundation Fact Sheet', National Headache Foundation, 2012, health-exchange.net/pdfdb/headfactEng.pdf

3   Senior, Kathryn, 'Facts and Figures About Headache'.

4   Alexander, Louise, 'Prevalence and Cost of Headache', *Headache Australia*, 2001, headacheaustralia.org.au/what-is-headache/11-prevalence-and-cost-of-headache

5   'WHO Report Ranks Migraine Among Top 20 Causes of Disability', *World Headache Alliance*, 28 February 2002, www.w-h-a.org/index.cfm/spKey/archive/spId/C1F71F9B-CEDC-7073-78E464689DD379E6.html

6   Collins, Lauren, 'Head First', *The New Yorker*, 21 September 2009.

7   Swan, Norman, 'Migraine Research', *Health Report*, ABC Radio National, 4 June 2012. Transcript available at www.abc.net.au/radionational/programs/healthreport/migraine-research/4039834

8   Kam, Katherine, 'Could Your Migraines Signal Uncontrolled Asthma?', *WebMD*, 22 June 2009, www.webmd.com/asthma/features/could-your-migraines-signal-uncontrolled-asthma

9   Cirillo, M., et al., 'Headache and Cardiovascular Risk Factors: positive association with hypertension', *Headache*, June 1999, no. 6, vol. 39, pp. 409–16, www.ncbi.nlm.nih.gov/pubmed/11279918

10 Visit Martin L. Pall's website at thetenthparadigm.org/index.html

11 The ME/CFS Society's website is www.mecfs.org.au; the AESSRA's website is www.aessra.org

12 For more information on this condition, visit en.wikipedia.org/wiki/

Sick_building_syndrome or www.patient.co.uk/doctor/Sick-Building-Syndrome.htm

13   Peterlin, B.L., et al., 'Migraine May Be a Risk Factor for the Development of Complex Regional Pain Syndrome', *Cephalalgia*, February 2012, vol. 30, no. 2, pp. 214–23, www.ncbi.nlm.nih.gov/pubmed/19614690

14   Green cited in Hughes, Sue, 'Migraine Increased in Coeliac and Inflammatory Bowel Disease', *Medscape*, 28 February 2013, www.medscape.com/viewarticle/780039

15   Mosher, Dave, 'Why Some Women Wear Too Much Perfume', *LiveScience*, 8 January 2008, www.livescience.com/2165-women-wear-perfume.html

16   Pall, Martin, *Explaining Unexplained Illnesses*, Haworth Press, 2007.

17   Jancin, Bruce, 'Migraine Called Major Risk Factor for Hyperemesis (Retrospective Study)', *OB GYN News*, December 2001, www.highbeam.com/doc/1G1-94158803.html

18   McCann, D., et al. 'Food Additives and Hyperactive Behaviour in 3-year-old and 8/9-year-old Children in the Community: a randomised, double-blinded, placebo-controlled trial', *Lancet*, 2007, pp. 1560–67.

19   This study is occurring at the Genomics Research Centre at Griffith University in Queensland, and other centres around the world.

20   Nurses Health Study, en.wikipedia.org/wiki/Nurses%27_Health_Study

21   Lea, Rod, et al., 'The Effects of Vitamin Supplementation and MTHFR (C677T) Genotype on Homocysteine-Lowering and Migraine Disability', *Pharmacogenetics and Genomics*, June 2009, vol. 19, no. 6, pp. 422–28.

22   Yasko, Amy, *Genetic Bypass*, Matrix Press, 2005, p. 51.

23   ibid.

24   Joshi, G., et al., 'Role of the ACE ID and MTHFR C677T Polymorphisms in Genetic Susceptibility of Migraine in a North Indian Population', *Journal of the Neurological Sciences*, vol. 277, no. 1, 15 February 2009, pp. 133–37. The Genomics Research Centre is also investigating this association.

25   Colson, N. J., et al., 'The Estrogen Receptor 1 G594A Polymorphism is Associated With Migraine Susceptibility in Two Independent Case/

Control Groups', *Neurogenetics*, vol. 5, no. 2, 2004, pp. 129–33; also the Genomics Research Centre.

26 Shearman, A., et al., 'Estrogen Receptor Alpha Gene Variation and the Risk of Stroke', *Stroke*, 2005, no. 36, pp. 22–81, American Heart Association, Inc., stroke.ahajournals.org/content/36/10/2281.short

27 Colson, N.J., et al., 'Investigation of Hormone Receptor Genes in Migraine', *Neurogenetics*, vol. 6, no. 1, February 2005, pp. 17–23, www.link.springer.com/journal/10048/6/1/page/1

28 'Migraine Cause "Identified" as Genetic Defect', *BBC News*, 27 September 2010, www.bbc.co.uk/news/health-11408113

29 Palotie, Aarno, 'First Genetic Link to Common Migraine Exposed', *Wellcome Trust Sanger Institute*, 29 August 2010, www.sanger.ac.uk/about/press/2010/100829.html. Doctor Palotie is chair of the International Headache Genetics Consortium at the Wellcome Trust Sanger Institute, which spearheaded the study.

30 'Research Uncovers Promising Target to Treat Chronic Abdominal Pain', *Ohio State University Research News*, March 2009, www.research-news.osu.edu/archive/viscpain.htm

31 Nyholt, Dale, et al., 'Evidence for an X-linked Genetic Component in Familial Typical Migraine', *Human Molecular Genetics*, vol. 7, no. 3, 1998, pp. 459–63, www.hmg.oxfordjournals.org/content/7/3/459.full.pdf

32 Lassen, L.H., et al., 'CGRP May Play a Causative Role in Migraine', *Cephalalgia*, vol. 22, no. 1, February 2002, pp. 54–61.

33 Luo, Xin-lin, et al., 'Association of CALCA Genetic Polymorphism With Essential Hypertension', *Chinese Medical Journal*, vol. 121, no. 15, 5 August 2008.

34 Ravilous, Kate, 'Mental Problems Gave Early Humans an Edge', *New Scientist*, 5 November 2011, p. 37.

35 'Serotonin Transporter', en.wikipedia.org/wiki/Serotonin_transporter

36 Egger, J., et al., 'Is Migraine Food Allergy? a double-blind controlled trial of oligoantigenic diet treatment', *Lancet*, vol. 2. no. 8355, 1983, pp. 86–59.

37 Munro, Jean, 'Food Allergy in Migraine', *Proceedings of the Nutrition Society*, vol. 42, 1983, p. 241.

38 Atkinson, W., et al., 'Food Elimination Based on IgG Antibodies in

Irritable Bowel Syndrome: a randomised controlled trial', *Gut*, vol. 53, 2004, pp. 1459–64, doi:10.1136/gut.2003.037697

39   The study was presented at the Third Congress of Headache Care for Practising Clinicians, Lisbon, Portugal, 1–3 October 2004, mipca.org. uk/pdf/HCPC_2004.pdf

40   Miller, Sheryl B., 'IgG Food Allergy Testing by ELISA/EIA: what do they really tell us?', *New Day Health*, www.newdayhealth.org/articles/ igg-food-allergy-testing.html

41   Pascual, Julio and Oterino, Augustin, 'IgG-mediated Allergy: a new mechanism for migraine attacks?' *Cephalalgia*, March 2010, doi:10.1177/0333102410364856

42   Discovered at Cornell University in 2003. See Kumar, Dhirendra and Klessig, Daniel F., 'High-affinity Salicylic Acid-binding Protein 2 is Required for Plant Innate Immunity and has Salicylic Acid-stimulated Lipase Activity', *Proceedings of the National Academy of Science USA*, vol. 100, 2003, pp. 16101–06.

43   Chen, Zhixiang and Klessig, Daniel F., 'Identification of a Soluble Salicylic Acid-binding Protein That May Function in Signal Transduction in the Plant Disease Resistance Responsem', *Proceedings of the National Academy of Science USA*, vol. 88, 1991, pp. 8179–83.

44   McCann, Donna, et al., 'Food Additives and Hyperactive Behaviour in 3-year-old and 8/9-year-old Children in the Community', *Lancet*, vol. 370, no. 9598, November 2007, pp. 1560–67.

45   ABC Radio National, *Health Report*, 4 June 2012, www.abc.net.au/radi-onational/programs/healthreport/migraine-research/4039834

46   Iannelli, Vincent, 'Motion Sickness', 17 August 2006, pediatrics.about. com/od/symptoms/a/0806_motionsick.htm

47   Drummond, Peter D. and Granston, Anna, 'Facial Pain Increases Nausea and Headache During Motion Sickness in Migraine Sufferers', *Brain*, March 2004, vol. 127, pt 3, pp. 526–34, www.ncbi.nlm.nih.gov/ pubmed/14749288

48   'Train Drivers Fall Ill From Safety Lights in New Tunnel', 7 July 2009, www.news.com.au/news/train-drivers-fall-ill-from-safety-lights-in-new-tunnel/story-fna7dq6e-1225746783651

49   Iqbal, Razia, 'Migraine Theory on Picasso Paintings', *BBC News*, 4
      September 2000, www.news.bbc.co.uk/2/hi/europe/909914.stm

50   'Fluorescent Lamps and Health', en.wikipedia.org/wiki/Fluorescent_
      lamps_and_health

51   Marcus, Caroline, 'Green Globes Trigger Mania', *Sydney Morning
      Herald*, 6 January 2008, www.smh.com.au/news/environment/green-
      globes-trigger-migraines/2008/01/05/1198950128815.html; Mayne,
      Eleanor, 'Energy-saving Light Bulbs "Are Threat to Epileptics"',
      The Daily Mail, 24 June 2007, http://www.dailymail.co.uk/health/
      article-463911/Energy-saving-light-bulbs-threat-epileptics.html. Also
      'Email to European Parliamentarians: low-energy light bulbs',
      www.groups.google.com/forum/#!msg/mobilfunk_newsletter/1JNPM_
      h9QSs/9dLf-jNycVYJ

52   Hecht, Jeff, 'Better Than Sunshine', *New Scientist*, 30 June 2012.

53   Hansen, Johnni, et al., 'Nested Case-control Study of Night Shift
      Work and Breast Cancer Risk Among Women in the Danish Military',
      Occupational and Environmental Medicine, May 2012, doi:10.1136/oemed-
      2011-100240:oem.bmj.com/content/early/2012/05/11/oemed-2011-
      100240; Holzman, David C., 'Blue Alert', *New Scientist*, 7 May 2011.

54   Gagnier, J. J., 'The Therapeutic Potential of Melatonin in Migraines
      and Other Headache Types', *Alternative Medicine Review*, August 2001,
      vol. 6, no. 4, pp. 383–39, www.ncbi.nlm.nih.gov/pubmed/11578254.
      See also www.medscape.com/viewarticle/488935

55   Kearney, Ray, 'Silent Smog — Electromagnetic Radiation', *ACNEM
      Journal*, vol. 29, no. 2, 2010.

56   Gagnier, J. J., 'The Therapeutic Potential of Melatonin in Migraines
      and Other Headache Types'.

57   Fragoso, Yara Dadalti, et al., 'Crying as a Precipitating Factor for
      Migraine and Tension-type Headache', *Sao Paulo Medical Journal*, 2003,
      vol. 121, no. 1, pp. 31–33, www.scielo.br/pdf/spmj/v121n1/16132.pdf

58   'Wind Turbines and Health: a rapid review of the evidence', National
      Health and Medical Research Council, July 2010, nhmrc.gov.au/_files_
      nhmrc/publications/attachments/new0048_evidence_review_wind_tur-
      bines_and_health.pdf

59   Ice-cream headache, en.wikipedia.org/wiki/Ice-cream_headache

60   Vein, A. A., et al., 'Space Headache: a new secondary headache',
      Cephalalgia, June 2009, vol. 29, no. 6, pp. 683–86, onlinelibrary.wiley.
      com/doi/10.1111/j.1468-2982.2008.01775.x/abstract

61   Phillips, Helen, 'Is Migraine All in the Mind?', *New Scientist*, 23 June 2003.

62   Kissela, Brett, 'Stroke Increasing at Younger Ages, UC Research
      Shows', University of Cincinnati, 24 February 2010, healthnews.
      uc.edu/news/?/9976/

63   Bercik, P., et al., 'The Anxiolytic Effect of *Bifidobacterium Longum*
      NCC3001 Involves Vagal Pathways for Gut–Brain Communication',
      Neurogastroenterology & Motility, December 2011, vol. 23, no. 12,
      pp. 1132–39.

64   McKie, Robin, 'Pain Relief "Cuts Heart Attack Victims' Survival
      Chances"', *Observer*, 8 April 2012. Also Naish, John, 'Stop Being a
      Wimp! Pain IS Good For You: how the dreaded sensation plays a cru-
      cial role in keeping us alive', *The Daily Mail*, 16 April 2012. Amadesi,
      Silvia, et al., 'Role for Substance P–Based Nociceptive Signaling in
      Progenitor Cell Activation and Angiogenesis During Ischemia in Mice
      and in Human Subjects?', *Circulation*, 2012, vol. 125, pp. 1774–86.

65   Strausbaugh, Holly J., 'Painful Stimulation Suppresses Joint
      Inflammation by Inducing Shedding of L-Selectin From Neutrophils',
      Nature Medicine, 1999, vol. 5, pp. 1057–61, doi:10.1038/12497

66   McCann, Donna, 'Food Additives and Hyperactive Behaviour in
      3-year-old and 8/9-year-old Children in the Community'.

67   Feingold Diet, en.wikipedia.org/wiki/Feingold_diet

68   *Julius Caesar*, act I, scene 2; *Othello*, act IV, scene 1 and act III, scene 3.

69   Gosline, Anna, 'Peanut Allergy: dining with death', *New Scientist*,
      June 2006, p. 40.

70   Kaulins, Andis, 'Human Blood Groups — Hybrid Modern Man',
      Lexiline: history of civilization, 20 June 2012, www.lexiline.com/lexiline/
      lexi9.htm

71   Lanou, Amy Joy, 'Bone Health in Children', *British Medical Journal*,
      October 2006, vol. 333, no. 7572, pp. 763–64, www.ncbi.nlm.nih.gov/
      pmc/articles/PMC1602030

72   Beaven, Michael A., 'Our Perception of the Mast Cell from Paul Ehrlich
      to Now', *European Journal of Immunology*, vol. 31, no. 1, January 2009,
      pp. 11–25, www.ncbi.nlm.nih.gov/pmc/articles/PMC2950100

73   Hegg, C. C., et al., 'Activation of Purinergic Receptor Subtypes
      Modulates Odor Sensitivity', *Journal of Neuroscience*, September 2003,
      vol. 23, no. 23, pp. 8291–301, www.ncbi.nlm.nih.gov/pubmed/12967991

74   Sherman, Paul W. and Flaxman, Samuel M., 'Protecting Ourselves
      from Food', *American Scientist*, March–April 2001, www.americanscien-
      tist.org/issues/feature/2001/2/protecting-ourselves-from-food

75   Motluck, Alison, 'Scent of a Man', *New Scientist*, 10 February 2001,
      www.motluk.com/stories/ns.scent.of.a.man.html

76   'Prohibited & Restricted Ingredients', *US Food and Drug
      Administration*, 30 May 2000, www.fda.gov/cosmetics/guidanceregula-
      tion/lawsregulations/ucm127406.htm#restricted

77   'Marketing Data: air-care market overview', *Star Candle*, 12 January
      2006, www.starcandle.com/report/MarketingReport.pdf

78   'Air Fresheners — A Global Strategic Business Report', Global
      Industry Analysts, Inc., April 2012, www.strategyr.com/Air_
      Fresheners_Market_Report.asp

79   Breyer, Melissa, 'Five Surprising Everyday Things That Are Toxic',
      Mother Nature Health Network, 24 April 2012, www.mnn.com/health/
      fitness-well-being/stories/5-surprising-everyday-things-that-are-toxic

80   Caress, S. M. and Steinemann, A. C., 'Prevalence of Fragrance
      Sensitivity in the American Population', *Journal of Environmental
      Health*, March 2009, vol. 71, no. 7, pp. 46–50.

81   Abrishami, Mohammad Hossein, 'Historical Background of Perfume
      and Perfume Manufacturing in Iran', *Iran Chamber Society*, www.iran-
      chamber.com/history/articles/historical_background_perfume_iran.
      php

82   'Perfume and Cologne', *Green Your: your guide to green living*,
      www.greenyour.com/body/cosmetics/perfume-and-cologne

83   Reiner, J. L., et al., 'Synthetic Musk Fragrances in Human Milk from
      the United States', *Environmental Science and Technology*, June 2007,
      vol. 41, no. 11, pp. 3815–20, www.ncbi.nlm.nih.gov/pubmed/17612154

84 Gilbère, Gloria, 'De-scents-itize Your Home/Office Part II', *TotalHealth Magazine*, 1 October 2012, www.totalhealthmagazine.com/articles/ environmental-health/de-scents-itize-your-home-office-part-ii.html; 'Prohibited & Restricted Ingredients', *US Food and Drug Administration*.

85 Kendall, Julia, '21 Most Common Chemicals Found in 31 Fragrance Products', *Mindfully.org*, 1993, www.mindfully.org/Pesticide/Fragrance-Product-Chemicals.htm. See also Lavelle, Peter, 'Not So Sweet: Chemicals in Fragrances', *ABC Health & Wellbeing*, 15 July 2010, www.abc.net.au/health/thepulse/stories/2010/07/15/2954502.htm; and 'Not So Sexy: the health risks of secret chemicals in fragrance', The Campaign for Safe Cosmetics, May 2010, www.safecosmetics.org/ article.php?id=644

86 Smith, Rick and Lourie, Bruce, *Slow Death by Rubber Duck*, University of Queensland Press, Brisbane, 2009, p. 4.

87 'With a Whiff of Eau de Baby', *Sydney Morning Herald*, 1 February 2013.

88 See some of those listed in 'Fragrance-free Policies', *My Chemical Fragrance-Free Life: the truth about toxic chemicals in commercial fragrances*, 2011, www.chemicalfragrancefree.wordpress.com/resources/ fragrance-free-policies; and 'Fragrance-free Organisations', *Nirvana Health*, www.nontoxic.com/nontoxic/scentfreeorganizations.html.

89 Bonk, Nancy Harris, 'Fragrance-free Campus', *Health Central*, 2007, www.healthcentral.com/migraine/c/202/15181/free-campus

90 Visit *ScentSense: all about fragrance* at www.scentsense.com.au

91 J.B, online comment on 'Migraine Research', *Health Report*, ABC Radio National, 4 June 2012, www.abc.net.au/radionational/programs/ healthreport/migraine-research/4039834

92 'Sweet Scent Doubles as Repellent for Flower Eaters', *New Scientist*, 9 December 2012, www.newscientist.com/article/mg21628944.700-sweet-scent-doubles-as-repellent-for-flower-eaters.html

93 Henley, Derek V., et al., 'Prepubertal Gynecomastia Linked to Lavender and Tea-tree Oils', *New England Journal of Medicine*, 2007, vol. 356, pp. 479–85.

94 'Multiple Chemical Sensitivities', *ME/CFS Australia (Victoria)*, 2011, www.mecfs-vic.org.au/multiple-chemical-sensitivities in Australia

95 Schoenen, Jean, et al., 'Effectiveness of High-dose Riboflavin in Migraine Prophylaxis: a randomized controlled trial', *Neurology*, vol. 50, no. 2, February 1998, pp. 466–70, www.neurology.org/content/50/2/466.short

96 Wang, Su-Jane, et al., 'Vitamin B2 Inhibits Glutamate Release From Rat Cerebrocortical Nerve Terminals', *Neuroreport*, vol. 19, no. 13, August 2008, pp. 1335–38, www.ncbi.nlm.nih.gov/pubmed/18695519

97 'Vitamin B2 Reduces Blood Pressure', *Food Product Design*, 18 February 2010, www.foodproductdesign.com/news/2010/02/vitamin-b2-reduces-blood-pressure.aspx

98 Simopoulos, A. P., 'The Importance of the Ratio of Omega-6/Omega-3 Essential Fatty Acids', *Biomedical Pharmacotherapy*, vol. 56, no. 8, October 2002, pp. 365–79, www.ncbi.nlm.nih.gov/pubmed/12442909

99 Small, Meredith F., 'The Happy Fat', *New Scientist*, 24 August 2002, www.newscientist.com/article/mg17523575.800-the-happy-fat.html

100 Tudge, Colin, *So Shall We Reap*, Penguin, London, 2003, p. 130.

101 Schattner, Peter, and Randerson, David, 'Tiger Balm as a Treatment of Tension Headache: a clinical trial in general practice', *Australian Family Physician*, vol. 25, no. 2, February 1996, pp. 216, 218, 220, www.ncbi.nlm.nih.gov/pubmed/8839380

102 Peikert, Andreas, et al., 'Prophylaxis of Migraine With Oral Magnesium: results from a prospective, multi-center, placebo-controlled and double-blind randomized study', *Cephalalgia*, vol. 16, no. 4, June 1996, pp. 257–63, www.onlinelibrary.wiley.com/doi/10.1046/j.1468-2982.1996.1604257.x/abstract

103 'Ajwain (Carom Seeds) Nutrition Facts', *Nutrition and You*, www.nutrition-and-you.com/ajwain.html

104 'Coenzyme Q10 May Stop Migraines', American Academy of Neurology, Annual Meeting, San Francisco, 28 April 2004, Abstract S43.004.

105 Cassels, Caroline, 'Vitamin D Deficiency Common in Patients with Chronic Migraine', American Headache Society 50th Annual Scientific Meeting, July 2008, www.medscape.com/viewarticle/577151

106 Mauskop, Alex, 'Blood Platelet Count and Migraines', 21 April 2011, www.migraine.com/blog/blood-platelet-count-and-migraines

107   Royal Pharmaceutical Society of Great Britain and British Medical Association, *British National Formulary*, Pharmaceutical Press, March 2011, London, p. 273.

108   Holmes, Bob, 'Is Coffee the Real Cure for a Hangover?' *New Scientist*, 11 January 2011, p. 17.

109   Jain, K. K., 'Triptans: clinical summary', *Medlink*, 9 June 2013, www.medlink.com/medlinkcontent.asp

110   Troost, B. T., 'Botulinum Toxin Type A (Botox) in the Treatment of Migraine and Other Headaches', *Expert Review of Neurotherapy*, vol. 4, no. 1, January 2004, pp. 27–31, www.ncbi.nlm.nih.gov/pubmed/15853612

111   Mathew, Ninan T., 'The Prophylactic Treatment of Chronic Daily Headache', *Headache: the journal of head and face pain*, vol. 46, no. 10, November–December 2006, pp. 1552–64.

112   Sun-Edelstein, C., and Mauskop, A., 'Alternative Headache Treatments: nutraceuticals, behavioral and physical treatments', *Headache*, vol. 51, issue 3, March 2011, pp. 469–83.

113   'Migraine', *National Health Service*, 14 May 2012, www.nhs.uk/conditions/Migraine/Pages/Introduction.aspx

114   Elkind, Arthur H., 'An Overview of Chronic Daily Headache', *Johns Hopkins Advanced Studies in Medicine*, vol. 6 (4D), April 2006, www.jhasim.net/files/articlefiles/pdf/ASM_6_4D_p325_330_R1.pdf

115   See Rea, William J., 'Inter-relationships Between the Environment and Premenstrual Syndrome', in Brush, M.G. and Goudsmit, E.M. (eds), *Functional Disorders of the Menstrual Cycle*, John Wiley and Sons, Chichester, 1988.

116   Geddes, Linda, 'Head Hurts? Zap the Wonder Nerve in Your Neck', *New Scientist*, 17 August 2013, www.newscientist.com/article/mg21929303.200-head-hurts-zap-the-wonder-nerve-in-your-neck.html

117   Elkind, 'An Overview of Chronic Daily Headache'.

118   Gorman, Christine, and Park, Alice, 'The New Science of Headaches'.

119   Haljamaue, H., and Hamberger, H., 'Potassium Accumulation by Bulk Prepared Neuronal and Glial Cells', *Journal of Neurochemistry*, vol. 18, no. 10, October 1971, pp. 1903–12, www.onlinelibrary.wiley.com/doi/10.1111/j.1471-4159.1971.tb09596.x/abstract

120 Rao, Shyam D., et al., 'Disruption of Glial Glutamate Transport by Reactive Oxygen Species Produced in Motor Neurons', *Journal of Neurosciences*, vol. 23, no. 7, 1 April 2003, pp. 2627–33.

121 Nahas, Stephanie, and Silberstein, Stephen, 'Triptans: Actions and Reactions', *Headache: the journal of head and face pain*, vol. 48, issue 4, pp. 611–13, April 2008, www.ncbi.nlm.nih.gov/pubmed/18377383

122 A potent clot-prevention drug, clopidogrel (brand name Plavix), is being tested in a clinical trial that will enrol nearly 300 migraine sufferers over three years. The trial is being run by John Chambers, a cardiologist at Guy's Hospital in London, who recently observed that the drug successfully cleared migraines in some of his patients — even those with no diagnosis of heart-valve defects. See also Moskowitz, Michael A., 'Cortical Spreading Depression is Key to Migraine Genesis', *Neurology Today*, vol. 7, no. 8, April 2007, pp. 42–43, www.aan.com/elibrary/neurologytoday/?event=home.showArticle&id=ovid.com:/bib/ovftdb/00132985-200704170-00016

123 Frietag, Fredrick G., 'Headache: advances in understanding and treatment', *The Lancet Neurology*, vol. 11, no. 1, pp. 10–12.

124 D'Andrea, Giovanni, et al., 'Biochemistry of Neuromodulation in Primary Headaches: focus on anomalies of tyrosine metabolism', *Neurological Sciences*, vol. 28, Supplement 2, May 2007, S94–S96.

125 Bartley, Jim, 'Case Study of Ms MT', *ACNEM Journal*, vol. 29, no. 2, September 2010, pp. 14–16.

126 ibid.

127 Dipalma, J. R., 'Tartrazine Sensitivity', *American Family Physician*, vol. 42, no. 5, November 1990, pp. 1347–50, www.ncbi.nlm.nih.gov/pubmed/2239641

128 Egger, J., et al., 'Is Migraine Food Allergy? a double-blind controlled trial of oligoantigenic diet treatment', *Lancet*, vol. 2, no. 8355, October 1983, pp. 865–69; Buist, Robert, *Food Chemical Sensitivity*, Harper & Row, Sydney, p. 46; Loblay, R. and Swain, A. R., 'Adverse Reactions to Tartrazine', *Food Technology in Australia*, vol. 37, 1985, pp. 508–10; Schab, D. W., et al., 'Do Artificial Food Colors Promote Hyperactivity in Children with Hyperactive Syndromes?: a meta-analysis of double-

blind placebo-controlled trials', *Developmental and Behavioral Pediatrics*, vol. 25, no. 6, December 2004, pp. 1560–67.

129 'Food Additives Altering Children's Behavior', *Better Health News and Comment*, vol. 2, number 8, www.thebetterhealthstore.com/news-letter/04-18_AprilNews02.html

130 Buist, *Food Chemical Sensitivity*, pp. 61, 84.

131 Browne, Rachel, 'Seeing Red Over Additives', *Sydney Morning Herald*, 26 September 2010, www.smh.com.au/lifestyle/diet-and-fitness/seeing-red-over-additives-20100925-15rkz.html

132 Buist, *Food Chemical Sensitivity*, p. 53.

133 European Food Safety Authority, *European Food Safety Authority Journal*, vol. 9, no. 1, 2011, pp. 1854–1900, www.efsa.europa.eu/en/efsajournal/pub/1854.htm

134 Littlewood, J. T., et al., 'Red Wine Contains a Potent Inhibitor of Phenolsulphotransferase', *British Journal of Clinical Pharmacology*, vol. 19, no. 2, February 1985, pp. 275–78.

135 Yasko, Amy, *Genetic Bypass*, Matrix Press, 2005, p. 79.

136 D'Andrea, Giovanni, et al., 'Platelet Levels of Dopamine are Increased in Migraine and Cluster Headache', *Headache: the journal of head and face pain*, vol. 46, no. 4, April 2006, pp. 585–91.

137 Melzig, M. F., et al., 'In Vitro Pharmacological Activity of the Tetrahydroisoquinoline Salsolinol Present in Products from Theobroma Cacao L. Like Cocoa and Chocolate', *Journal of Ethnopharmacology*, vol. 73, nos. 1–2, November 2000, pp. 153–59.

138 Flechas, J. D., 'Iodine and the Body', *Iodine Research: resource network of the iodine movement*, www.iodineresearch.com/breastpg2.html

139 Li, Mu, et al., 'Are Australian Children Iodine Deficient?: results of the Australian National Iodine Nutrition Study', *Medical Journal of Australia*, vol. 184, no. 4, 2006, pp. 165–69, www.mja.com.au/journal/2006/184/4/are-australian-children-iodine-deficient-results-australian-national-iodine

140 McKendrick, Allison M. et al., 'Visual and Auditory Perceptual Rivalry in Migraine', *Cephalalgia*, vol. 31, no. 11, August 2011, pp. 1158–69, www.cep.sagepub.com/content/31/11/1158

141 Houle, Timothy T., 'Not Tonight, I Have a Headache?', *Headache: the journal of head and face pain*, 2006, vol. 46, no. 6, pp. 983–90, www.archive/shj3L

142 Beagle, Bill, 'Aspartame is Neurotoxic Genotoxid Molecular Food and Vaccine Pharmaco-genocide', *Whale*, www.whale.to/b/deagle_asp.html

143 Giffin, N. J., 'Paroxysmal Hemicrania by GTN', *Cephalalgia*, vol. 27, August 2007, pp. 953–54.

144 Lea, Rod, et al., 'The Effects of Vitamin Supplementation and MTHFR (C677T) Genotype on Homocysteine-lowering and Migraine Disability', *Pharmacogenetics and Genomics*, vol. 19, no. 6, June 2009, pp. 422–28, www.researchgate.net/publication/24346408_The_effects_of_vitamin_supplementation_and_MTHFR_(C677T)_genotype_on_homocysteine-lowering_and_migraine_disability/file/79e415063a52f0dad6.pdf

145 Hohoff, C., et al., 'An Adenosine A2A Receptor Gene Haplotype is Associated with Migraine with Aura', *Cephalalgia*, vol. 27, no. 2, February 2007, pp. 177–81, www.cep.sagepub.com/content/27/2/177.abstract

146 Sicuteri, F., and Nicolodi M., 'Exploration of NMDA Receptors in Migraine: therapeutic and theoretic implications', *International Journal of Clinical Pharmacology Resources*, vol. 15, no. 5–6, 1995, pp. 181–89, www.ncbi.nlm.nih.gov/pubmed/8835616; Hohoff, 'An Adenosine A2A Receptor Gene Haplotype is Associated with Migraine with Aura'.

147 Hamilton, Garry, 'Filthy Friends and the Rise of Allergies', *New Scientist*, 16 April 2005, www.newscientist.com/article/mg18624951.900-filthy-friends-and-the-rise-of-allergies.html

148 Shi, G. X., et al., 'Toll-like Receptor Signaling Alters the Expression of Regulator of G Protein Signaling Proteins in Dendritic cells: implications for G-protein-coupled receptor signaling', *Journal of Immunology*, vol. 172, 2004, pp. 5175–84.

149 Bartley, Jim , 'Case Study of Ms MT', *ACNEM Journal*, September 2010, vol. 29, no. 2, pp. 14–16.

150 Tang, C. M., 'Genetic Variation in G-protein-coupled Receptors: consequences for G-protein-coupled receptors as drug targets', *Expert Opinion on Therapeutic Targets*, vol. 9, no. 6, December 2005, pp. 1247–65, www.ncbi.nlm.nih.gov/pubmed/16300474

151 Jane C Figueiredo et al, 'Folic Acid and Risk of Prostate Cancer: results from a randomized clinical trial', *Journal of the National Cancer Institute*, vol. 101, no. 6, 2009, pp. 432–435, doi:10.1093/jnci/djp019

152 Mestel, Rosie, 'Feeling a Little Strange', *New Scientist*, 14 June 1997, pp. 24–28.

Index